NIGHT
REFLECTIONS

NIGHT
REFLECTIONS

A True Story of Friendship, Love, Cancer, and Survival

ROBERT T. WINN, M.D.

WITH

TIMOTHY R. PEARSON

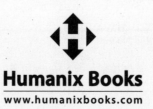

Humanix Books

www.humanixbooks.com

Humanix Books

Night Reflections: A True Story of Friendship, Love, Cancer, and Survival
Copyright © 2016 by Humanix Books
All rights reserved

Humanix Books, P.O. Box 20989, West Palm Beach, FL 33416, USA
www.humanixbooks.com I info@humanixbooks.com

Library of Congress Cataloging-in-Publication Data

Names: Winn, Robert Thomas, author.
Title: Night reflections : a true story of friendship, love, cancer, and
    survival / Robert Thomas Winn, MD.; with Timothy R. Pearson.
Description: West Palm Beach, FL : Humanix Books, [2016]
Identifiers: LCCN 2016017794 (print) I LCCN 2016029922 (ebook) I
    ISBN 9781630060701 (hardback) I ISBN 9781630060718 (ebook) I
    ISBN 9781630060442 (e-book)
Subjects: LCSH: Winn, Robert Thomas, Health. I Leukemia—Patients—
    Biography—Utah. I Cancer—Patients—Utah—Biography. I Leukemia—
    Patients—Family relationships. I Husband and wife. I BISAC: HEALTH
    & FITNESS / Diseases / Cancer. I HEALTH & FITNESS / Women's
    Health.
Classification: LCC RC643 .W546 2016 (print) I LCC RC643 (ebook) I
    DDC 616.99/4190092 [B]—dc23
LC record available at https://lccn.loc.gov/2016017794

Cover photo: Getty Images 186837005
Interior design: Scribe Inc.

Humanix Books is a division of Humanix Publishing, LLC. Its trademark,
consisting of the words "Humanix" is registered in the Patent and Trademark
Office and in other countries.

ISBN: 978-1-63006-070-1 (Hardcover)
ISBN: 978-1-63006-071-8 (E-book)

Printed in the United States of America
10 9 8 7 6 5 4 3 2 1

Dedication

To the countless patients and their families who have battled cancer together; to the many gifted researchers who have persistently advanced the science of treating leukemia; to the devoted staff of the trio of hospitals in which my beloved Nancy spent the better part of a year; to my late mother, who taught me the ideals that led to my own career in medicine, showed me how to unearth the goodness in others, and exposed me to the beauty and power of the written word; and finally, to the anonymous donor who altruistically gifted his bone marrow to Nancy and, in so doing, gave her a chance at life.

Contents

Foreword

A diagnosis of acute myeloid leukemia is a shocking, disorienting, terrifying event. Only a month ago, your life was unfolding as usual. Only one week ago, you sensed something wasn't quite right, noticing just a bit more fatigue and a few unexpected bruises. Only a minute ago, you heard your doctor declare that you have leukemia. Without therapy, you are told that you will likely die in a few weeks and that the only alternative is to receive intensive chemotherapy—which itself could kill you. If, following initial therapy, you are fortunate enough to enter a complete remission, you are advised that you will need further treatment to keep the leukemia from recurring. Later, you will have to make a decision between receiving additional chemotherapy versus undergoing a bone marrow transplant, one of the most crucial and anxiety-producing decisions in all of clinical medicine. Simply, it could happen to any of us, and it did to Nancy Winn.

In *Night Reflections*, Robert Winn, himself a physician, describes the roller coaster events following his wife's diagnosis of acute myeloid leukemia. The book is medically and scientifically accurate. More importantly, Dr. Winn's story is remarkably open, unguarded, and intimate—a personal journey of discovery, friendship, love, and ultimately survival. Dr. Winn's willingness to candidly explore and expose his own vulnerabilities provides an honest look into the tumultuous and sometimes chaotic events experienced by a caring husband and family as a loved one faces a potentially fatal illness. I believe that almost any physician, staff member, patient, patient family member, or friend will come away with new insights and understanding after reading this moving memoir.

Nancy Winn was blessed to have a supportive husband and family. She was also fortunate to be treated in the current era rather than a few decades ago. Medical advances have been significant in many ways. Although the treatment of acute myeloid leukemia still leaves much to be desired, there has been noteworthy recent improvement in outcomes. Today, the risk of dying from a complication of chemotherapy has dropped remarkably, mostly due to the development of better ways to combat infection. With this advance and the development of new chemotherapies and refinements in their use, cure rates with chemotherapy alone have increased from 15% to almost 50%. Outcomes with bone marrow transplantation have likewise improved over the last several decades, and cure rates of 65% are now regularly reported. The credit for these advances goes to the scientists and clinicians who developed and tested these new approaches. But enormous credit should also be given to the countless patients who willingly participated in the clinical trials that were required to test these new approaches and demonstrate their effectiveness.

Nancy Winn did not have a matched sibling to serve as a donor but rather received her transplant from an unrelated volunteer donor. The first transplant from a matched unrelated donor was reported in 1980. It was obvious from the very beginning that if unrelated transplants were to become widely available, a very large donor registry would have to be created. Remarkably, today over 25 million normal individuals have agreed to be typed and entered into an international registry to provide bone marrow for individuals they have never met and to do so for no financial or other reward. While Nobel prizes and honorary degrees go to leading scientists and clinicians, there are many other heroes in the fight against leukemia, including past patients, volunteer donors and societies, and supportive, loving family members like the Winns.

Frederick R. Appelbaum, MD
Director, Clinical Research Division,
Fred Hutchinson Cancer Research Center
Head, Division of Oncology,
University of Washington School of Medicine
President, Seattle Cancer Care Alliance in Seattle, Washington

Acknowledgments

When my wife, Nancy, was diagnosed with an aggressive form of acute myeloid leukemia, our lives changed forever. Overnight, our world went from the normality of daily life to one tumbling and careening out of control. For the next two years, we existed under the dark uncertainty of a life-threatening disease and amid the roller coaster of tests, treatments, and hospitals. My escape was my medical practice, and my only comfort was the unwavering support of our families, friends, and our community. Heartbreakingly, I simply began to cry whenever I was asked about Nancy.

Since it was so much easier for me to write than to talk, I began composing letters on many of the evenings that I sat quietly and resolutely beside my acutely ill wife in the soft, flickering nighttime lights of her hospital room. My middle-of-the-night updates became the way for me to share our journey with our friends and family. And over time, I came to learn that these late-night reflections depicting our struggles and travails touched the hearts of friends and acquaintances alike.

Critically, scores of our friends reassured me that it was all right to communicate with them during these hours of darkness. Their constant caring and expressions of encouragement allowed me to share my most intimate thoughts and fears. Without this positive feedback and overwhelming acceptance, I would not have continued my writings during those two years. To them, I will forever and always be grateful.

Shortly after Nancy's final hospitalization, I received a very special gift from Edgar and Polly Stern, longtime friends of ours. Polly had saved each of my middle-of-the-night letters and compiled them into a compendium she titled *A Love Story: Letters from Winnie*. When I was given the twenty-five copies that Polly had self-published, she said, "At some point, your loved ones will want to read this story. It's important. And you should consider sharing your words with others." Polly possessed a gentle kindness and a gigantic heart. Her gift reflected her person: Caring. Insightful. Inspiring. Little did I know how important her gift would become—because I had not saved any of my writings.

Since then, a similar sentiment has often been expressed to me. Yet for many all-too-self-apparent reasons, I was always hesitant to revisit and retrace our journey, because to do so was simply too painful. But with the passage of time, I healed, too. The tipping point for me came at a most unexpected time and surprising place.

Late last year, near the end of the ski season, I was at a small, intimate dinner party in a mountain yurt on the upper slopes of the Canyons Ski Resort in Park City, Utah. Unexpectedly, I ran into Kristin Barber, who I hadn't seen since she had been a nurse practitioner student in our office. She said, "Winnie, I've been wanting to tell you something important. You had an impact on my life." She explained that she had asked to be on my mailing list and that my writings had influenced her career choice—she became an oncology nurse practitioner. Like Polly, Kristin proclaimed, "I hope you will publish your writings someday for others to learn from and find inspiration—just like I did."

By sheer coincidence, Tim Pearson, a close friend and the brother of Tom Pearson, the two hosts of the evening's affair (and himself an author who had written the critically acclaimed *New York Times* bestseller *The Old Rules are Dead*), had been talking with Kristin before my arrival. He listened thoughtfully to our exchange. "Would you like to publish your letters?" he asked. "Send me copies. I'll give you my honest opinion and offer some suggestions on where to go with a manuscript."

I don't know if it was the wine, the circumstances, or both. I sent one of Polly's compilations to Tim the next day. The rest, as they say, is history. With his unwavering, nurturing guidance and rigorous editing, *Love Letters from Winnie* was transformed into *Night Reflections: A True Story of Friendship, Love, Cancer, and Survival.* Our chance meeting led to both his ongoing sage counsel and his truly invaluable continuing involvement that challenged and sustained my efforts during our own journey of discovery together. This book is his as much as it is mine.

Author's Note

Quite simply, I have always lived more in my head than in my heart. As a pediatrician and the longtime medical leader of both the Deer Valley Resort and the Park City Mountain Resort on-mountain medical teams, my early childhood predisposition and affinity to science (and ultimately medicine) has served me well. I have treated literally thousands of patients over the years. And I consider myself privileged to have been able to provide both care and consolation to those in need of my skills and talents.

On any given day, I can be faced with life-and-death decisions that require not only an understanding of human nature but also a vast encyclopedic knowledge of standard protocols, complex procedures, prescriptive approaches, and surgical outcomes. My decisions are carefully considered, patient centered, and caringly advocated. My patient's lives literally depend on me. And there simply isn't any room for errors in my chosen line of work. (Or, for that matter, any practicing or attending physician. I am no different.)

I was born in what seems like a very different world than the one that we live in today. Penn's Woods (or Pennsylvania for those not a product of the suburbs south of Philadelphia) was a simpler, more rural place than it is now. My parents were very "old school" and married after a short courtship when my mother was in her early twenties and my father was in his mid-thirties.

My mother was vivacious and a model of openness. She expressed her feelings clearly, honestly, and frankly. She possessed an ability to describe and illuminate the solution to almost any problem. And she naturally and freely displayed her emotions.

When my father died after a protracted and grueling battle with cancer, she was left to raise two children, and I was left at an early age to be the "man of the house." This tumultuous time period transformed me, and I increasingly found ever-greater comfort in ideas, equations, books—as well as the quiet outdoors, where I could be surrounded by the smells, sounds, and wonders of nature.

As an adult, I have changed over time, but it wasn't until I met and married Nancy that I truly became the man and husband that I am now. She changed my life. She changed my world. Simply, Nancy changed me in such a way that I could never again live as a man divided.

This is our story—a tale of despair, of love, and ultimately of survival. And, like all stories, it has a beginning—one that, for me, begins with the change of the seasons.

Prelude

As ski season ends in the Rockies, a jagged range of geologically complex mountains partially covered by glaciers and high peaks that I have called home for over forty-one years, snow still abounds in any direction the eyes pivot. Unfailingly, year in and year out, as April dissolves into May, frequent storms unleash walls of rain rather than the wondrous white offerings dumped with great abandon during winter. Colored rooftops quickly emerge from beneath what is always, for that time of year, still a thick blanket of winter snow.

In contrast, the lower elevations cling only to those last few white patches that are both north-facing and protected by tree shadows. The sun, which ascends ever upward into the sky, consistently raises the temperatures above freezing during most daylight hours. With each passing day, the snow retreats higher and higher up the ski runs toward the mountaintops while the water released by such rapid melting turns the ground beneath into vast archipelagoes of dark, thick, heavy mud.

Unlike summer when the mountains are clothed in green grass and matching foliage, or fall when they burst into an audacious display of yellow aspen and red Rocky Mountain maple leaves, or winter, of course, with the entire landscape carpeted in pristine white snow, spring "mud season" is the solitary time of year that I have learned over the years to describe with a singular and simple declaration—*Ugh!*

Annually, the mud on the ground blends unobtrusively with the browns and grays of the leafless trees and the still-slumbering ground cover. The faint fresh scent of winter pine needles is replaced by the strong, musty smell of old shoes. During this desolate and lonely time of year, the mountains are uninviting; they seem filled with decay. Some of the older trees have been toppled, some of the bushes appear damaged beyond recovery, and the many trails are nearly impossible to navigate. Mud cakes to anything that dares step on it and at the very worst imitates quicksand that will swallow a shoe failing to tread lightly.

With the prized jewel of mountain living tarnished by this once-a-year transition, I annually experience misery and gloom as reoccurring daily emotions rather than the hope and optimism that are my normal daily companions. Mud season, for some unplumbed and unknown reason, always elicits threatening, foreboding, and ominous feelings in the core of my being.

Unlike the rest of the year, when bright sunshine or sparkling snow cover lifts my spirits, many days are overcast with nondescript gray clouds that intermittently spew a dull drizzle. Inexplicably, I am often left with the disconsolate heartache of melancholy. No wonder that the local schools celebrate a nine-day spring break, many restaurants and businesses lock their doors for a week or so, and anybody with the time and the wherewithal ventures south to escape the mud and its resulting dark mindset.

Mud season reminds me that even in a mountain paradise there can be days and weeks when nature's turmoil can cast off her customary beauty, when fresh smells can turn sour, when brilliance can fade to dreariness. I can close the shades in my office and ignore its existence; I can flee my home to an alternate place and pretend mud season doesn't exist; I can bravely trudge through the dense, black, glutinous earth until it makes my shoes so heavy they can't endure another step. What I can't do is change a fundamental truth.

Mud season is part of the never-ending cycle of nature.

Every spring, the change in seasons forces me to think about mortality and rebirth because near the end of May, the mountains vividly reclaim their magnificence. Overnight, buds appear on the Saskatoon serviceberry, the narrowleaf cottonwood, and the many other trees that, like me, call the mountains home. The new growth provides a pleasing contrast with the abundant Gamble oak trees, whose twisted branches and trunks always remain naked at least until June.

Wild grasses will soon reclaim wooded areas and open fields and, like the needles on the Rocky Mountain junipers, Douglas fir, and Engelmann spruce trees that dot the mountains in mini-forests, sport a glittering sheen, having been thoroughly rinsed of any winter debris by the recent spring downpours. Shoots of bluebells, larkspurs, and sticky geraniums explode through the drying earth to impart a dazzling array of colors that rival the frequent rainbows that always accompany the last of the big rains. A camphor-like odor from the plentiful sagebrush is the most pungent smell among a luminous mix of fragrances.

Birds are suddenly ubiquitous, with northern mockingbirds chirping, blue grosbeaks singing, and male American robins chasing each other from tree to tree. Sightings of Shiras moose and mule and white-tailed deer proliferate, not because the animals are returning to the mountains, but rather because the weather stabilizes and, more likely than not, it will be sunny. With the mud quickly drying, the town residents and I reemerge late each spring to utilize the many trails without risk of ruining a new pair of sneakers or hiking boots.

The passing of mud season is like the reoccurring dawn following the darkness, the all too quiet after the storm, or the miraculous birth of a newborn. When mud season ends, the uncharacteristic and ever-present feelings that have haunted me during the frozen winter months quickly disappear. I recover and my mood always swiftly brightens, bordering on euphoria like a resilient fighter battling and overcoming insurmountable odds.

Hope, with the life-changing knowledge that spring will turn to summer, is everything.

The Beginning

On the last day of May, Kathleen Thomas, my partner at the Park City Family Health Center, was eagerly waiting for me when I arrived at the trailhead of Glenwild, a private golf community set amid the expansive, flower-filled meadows and majestic alpine slopes in Park City, Utah. Excitedly, Kathleen, or "KT" as she was known by her friends, and I were about to embark on our first mountain bike outing of the year, and I was surprised that she had beaten me there because I was, as is my custom, early. (Kathleen's clock usually runs about fifteen minutes behind everyone else's.)

"I'm *soooo* motivated, Winnie!" she yelled as I opened my car door. "But we'll need to go slow since I'm not in shape yet."

Kathleen, forty-five years old and fourteen years my junior, was being modest. In reality, she is in better shape than most people I know. She was a college athlete and is still trim, possessing a runner's physique. She can talk incessantly while she pedals even on the steepest inclines, while I have difficulty answering "Uh Huh" or "No" to her many questions and breathing at the same time. I was relieved to hear the pace wouldn't be too aggressive.

We unloaded our respective Giant Anthem full-suspension mountain bikes, grabbed our Camelbak M.U.L.E. hydration backpacks, and steered up the trail. Unlike our much longer rides later in the season, it would be a forty-minute ascent to the summit, much of it switchbacks at a reasonable grade with only a few steep sections requiring our lowest gear and our highest energy.

"I don't think we'll need our 'blueies' long, Winnie," she declared. "It's really warming up."

Kathleen has lots of names for things. "Blueies" are the blue windbreaker shells we utilize for warmth and rain protection. The temperature, a chilly forty-four degrees, made our ears and noses tingle as we left the parking lot. It was only 10:35 a.m. and the thermometer was already rising faster than the climbing sun. The effort required for the uphill leg of the journey would certainly produce extra heat.

"Sounds good," I replied. "Let's pedal for ten minutes and then take a break so we can shed our outer shells."

Frankly, to be back on my bike was glorious. We rapidly left the parking area and with each successive switchback faced a more commanding view of the scenery below. The entire valley, christened the Snyderville Basin by the Utah pioneers, was encircled by the majestic backside of the Wasatch Mountains, a north-to-south range that defines the western edge of the Rocky Mountains. Nestled snugly into the base of the distant peaks to our right was "Old Town," once a silver mining community and now the cultural center of Park City. Distinct clusters of homes extended toward us like the spokes of a wheel.

Despite the explosive growth over the nearly three decades that I have lived in the area, much of what we viewed remained open space. A patchwork of gentle farmland displayed squares alternately tan, green, or gold reflecting crops of alfalfa, hay, and triticale that would soon be as high as an adult's waist. Small clumps of quaking aspen and Douglas fir trees, sitting like islands in a sea of homes, provided additional space that was undeveloped. But the most impressive and vast expanse of untouched beauty comprised the alternately smooth and jagged tops of the distant mountains. Fortunately, neither homes nor development had ventured to that elevation. The still white-capped peaks blended splendidly with a sky the light-blue color of the Mediterranean Sea.

Puffy wisps of clouds dotted the sky, and among the many shapes and sizes were a towering giant holding a big stick, the upper half of a dolphin leaping from the ocean, and the lateral view of a woman's face as angular as my riding partner Kathleen's. The breathtaking panorama alone validated the considerable effort required to push uphill.

With crisp air that smelled as fresh as newly washed laundry, my breathing rate increased as we ascended skyward. To our surprise and delight, the entire trail was dry and without the ruts that appear after heavy use. Under these ideal conditions, mastering the roots and rocks only added to the enjoyment of the first bike adventure of the riding season.

On both sides of the trail, the Bitterbrush trees were teeming with buds and ripening blueberries. In all directions, we were greeted by the first wild flowers of the season. Tall clumps of yellow arrowleaf balsamroot stood guard over delicate yellow glacier lilies. Vast expanses of lavender and plum mountain daisies lined many stretches of our track. An entire field of tiny blue forget-me-nots swayed lazily in the breeze. And an orange flower whose name escaped me nestled beside the first Indian paintbrush. I was hypnotized by its bright-red hue. In those sections of the trail that had been cut into the mountain leaving a ledge, the clematis vines dangled tentacles strung with large purple flowers that shimmered in the sun like Christmas tree lights.

It was hard to not run off our winding dirt trail because too much attention was being paid to the surrounding splendor and too little to the ground in front of our wheels. As we reached the top and laid our bikes down for a well-deserved snack of M&M's and pretzel mini-sticks, I took an extra deep breath that was not the result of exertion. Even though my hands throbbed a little and a small twinge of discomfort in my lower back reminded me that I was not a teenager, there was no doubt—this was a *perfect* day.

Resting on a verdant knoll well suited for our little resting place, the grass was soft to the touch. I pulled a long blade and dangled it in my mouth like a country boy on a farm, even though I had been born in the suburbs of Philadelphia. For a while, Kathleen and I talked as only longtime friends can about kids, medicine, and the mundane details of life. Refreshed, we stood and absorbed our summiting accomplishment before slapping hands in a triumphant high five and prepared to re-saddle for the blissfully easy trip back down. Startlingly, the moment was interrupted by the sound of a harp emanating from my mobile phone, the screen revealing a familiar number and an even more familiar image—Nancy, my wife and best friend. In her job as a flight attendant, Nancy was on a three-day trip back East.

"Hi, Winnie. Sorry to disturb your bike ride." The previous night, before going to bed in Cleveland, Nancy had asked during our routine daily good-night conversation about my plans for my day off. She had been pleased I would be enjoying my favorite outdoor passion.

"No bother. KT and I are at the summit and about to head down. What's up?"

Nancy and I had been married for twenty-seven years. Though I encouraged otherwise, she was generally loath to call me at work or at play. I detected some concern in her voice, which troubled me. Blood flushed my face slightly and the sweat on my hands was no longer entirely from exertion.

"On my flight this morning, I had a nosebleed. It stopped in a few moments, but I'm at the hotel now in Boston and it's started again. What should I do?"

As a primary care physician for over thirty years, I have treated countless patients with nosebleeds. But hearing this particular news gave me an inexplicably peculiar feeling deep in my stomach. Instead of merely telling Nancy how to squeeze her nose or how to pack it with Kleenex, I asked additional questions.

"Is the bleeding on one side of your nose or both?"

"Have you been sick at all?"

"Do you have a fever or chills?"

"Do you have a rash?"

And so on . . .

When I finally hung up, Kathleen asked, "What's up? You seem more concerned than I'd expect you to be for a simple nosebleed." Kathleen was the most gifted nurse practitioner I knew. She was my daughter's primary care provider.

"I must be a little tired from our climb, and I'm worried for some reason. I honestly don't know why."

Goosebumps crept up my arms even though the ambient temperature was now quite comfortable. Like many doctors, I possess an extra "sense" that sometimes gives me pause. My intuition is often potent and instinctive.

Just the week before, a longtime friend had come into the office with a common everyday complaint—a bad headache. Stan had not scheduled a doctor's visit in five years, and as a stoic lifelong rancher who had been thrown off his horse more times than I had ridden one, he once told me, "Don't like doctors much, Winnie. No offense." Stan wouldn't have been sitting on my exam table unless the headache was really bad, though you wouldn't have known it based on the look on his face or the sound of his voice.

Instead of trying symptomatic care when his medical history didn't raise any red flags and his neurologic exam was normal, I uncharacteristically decided to send him immediately for a CAT scan. Something in the pit of my stomach told me this was the right decision. He was admitted to the hospital as soon as the test was completed and had brain surgery that same evening. The neurosurgeon told him later that the cerebral aneurism was ready to rupture at any moment.

"Nancy will be fine, Winnie. It's probably the dry airplane air. Didn't she have a cold last week? Maybe she had a scab inside her nose break loose."

Riding a mountain bike downhill is exhilarating. The challenge is not cardiovascular as it is on the way up; rather it is skill based. Which rocks to avoid and which ones to simply jump over while letting your hands and the bike's shock absorb the bumps is mandatory know-how. Proficiency is crucial. A good rider knows how to lean into a sharp turn without wiping out and when to slow down to avoid a serious fall.

Kathleen and I have a shared and long-held mantra—no blood. We are pretty conservative riders compared to many of Park City's younger mountain bikers. Still, after a long climb, the downhill leg is normally an unadulterated thrill ride—one that harkens back to the feeling I had when I dismounted my first roller coaster as a seven-year-old, screaming in complete joy to my waiting mother, "That was fun! Wow!" Even today, the memory makes my face hurt from a too-wide smile.

I had been so looking forward to the well-earned return to the parking area, but the twenty-minute descent was anticlimactic. The gnawing in my gut persisted. Instead of enjoying the wind whipping through my hair, the thrill of successfully mastering the bumps and curves, and the companionship of one of my best friends, I was preoccupied. I couldn't shake my thoughts of Nancy. A scab letting loose couldn't have caused the problem. The nosebleed was on both sides.

For nearly an hour after my arrival back at the trailhead where I had parked the car, I waited uneasily. I paced around the car like an expecting father in a delivery room. I spun my bike pedals backward again and again just to hear the click-click-click sound that was always music to my ears.

Finally, I dialed the number I know as well as my own. Nancy answered in one ring. "You were right, Winnie. I squeezed my nose. Five straight minutes by the clock. It did the trick." She added that she felt "absolutely fine," would get a good night's sleep, and would see me tomorrow in the early evening.

Nonetheless, after Kathleen and I said our good-byes and I returned home late in the day, the sheep in my suddenly all-too-empty bedroom were out in flocks. I felt drained and exhausted, though not from the day's activity. It was a restless, uneasy sleep that night.

The next day, my riding partner was another good friend, Chuck English, the director of mountain operations at Deer Valley Resort. During the winters, we worked together very closely because I was the medical director for the resort. And in the nonski- and nonmud-season months, we rode together two or three times a week. I was also his family's primary care physician.

The day was nearly a carbon copy of my outing with Kathleen. We did the identical ride, Glenwild, because it was still the only major Park City trail that was entirely dry. After another classic spring excursion, as we were strapping our bikes to the back of my car, my phone made the familiar harp sound.

"Nancy, how are you? Did your nose bleed last night?"

"I'm fine, Winnie. I hate to bother you again before you get home. Are you still with Chuck?"

"I am, but no worries. What's going on?"

"Remember you asked me if I had a rash? I was dressing this morning for today's trip, and when I looked in the mirror, I do have a rash."

"Where is it, Nancy?"

"Pretty much all over—especially on my arms and legs. On my left thigh, it looks like a bruise. And I don't remember running into anything."

"Have you had another nosebleed?"

"Well, a few times. But it always stops with pressure. I don't feel sick, and I know I don't have a fever. What should I do?"

"I think you should go to a doctor right now. You may have to miss your flight."

"I can't do that, Winnie. There's no one to replace me. I'm actually on my way to the airport right now. I only work a few legs and should be home by early evening. I can see someone tomorrow if you really think it's necessary."

Twenty-seven years together. Whether it was our marriage, the kids, her many friends, or her job, Nancy was all about two things: dedication and commitment. Though I felt warmth in my heart, I felt tightness in my chest. I knew this was an argument I wouldn't win.

"Fine, I guess. Call me as soon as you land in Salt Lake. You may need to go the emergency room once you get here."

"Don't be such a worrywart. I'm fine. I love you."

"I love you, too."

After turning away from Chuck, I wiped the tears that were beginning to drop down my cheeks with the back of my hand. When I turned back toward Chuck, he looked at me and immediately asked, "Are you okay, Winnie?"

My profession as a practicing family doctor has many wonderful positive qualities, including the ability to help others and to be an essential part of their lives, the academic challenge and pure delight of never-ending learning, the reality that my medical expertise provides reasonable compensation for me and my family, and the freedom to work almost anywhere in the world. However, like it or not, there is a very real negative that is a doctor's recurring reality: sometimes you know too much. And this was one of those times.

As I looked upward to the mountain I had just traversed, the colors didn't seem nearly as bright. My parking lot vantage point revealed more Gamble oak trees waiting for leaves than all the other trees already dressed in olive, jade, and emerald. The flowers and grasses were no longer visible, and there was more brown and gray than when I had been up at the summit. A cloud now covered the sun, and the sky had lost its luster. A sudden chill seized the air and I unthinkingly rubbed both arms for warmth. As the sky darkened with the threat of rain, I irrationally wondered, *"Could mud season be returning?"*

NIGHT
REFLECTIONS

As Sick as a Person Can Be

May 30, 4:13 a.m.

Dear Family,

I am writing you in the late hours of darkness with a heavy heart after an utterly sleepless night. At the moment, I am an emotional cripple, unable to talk to anyone, even a stranger. So I apologize for using this group letter to communicate. An all-too-brief and impersonal communication will have to suffice until I don't burst into tears every time I try to talk. Sadly, we are anxiously awaiting the confirmatory tests, but there is every indication that Nancy has the blood cancer called leukemia.

Last night, Nancy was admitted to LDS Hospital in Salt Lake City. Her skin was hot and the thermometer reading topped at 105.2 degrees. Purple bruises covered much of her body due to a deficiency of platelets, the type of blood cell responsible for clotting. The red oxygen-carrying blood cells were so severely depleted that Nancy's blood count was barely more than half of normal, meaning she was quite anemic. And, hardest for me to witness, the bright aura that normally surrounds my bride's demeanor seemed dimmed to a mere flicker.

Though her radiant smile retained its warmth, her normally gentle forehead lines were pulled tight with discomfort and her speech was flat and barely audible. In fact, the only words Nancy uttered loud enough for me to discern were, "Don't say anything to the kids yet, Winnie. I don't want Jaret and Jayna to worry." As I held both of her hands and put my ear close to her mouth, all other sentences were just mumbles. She was in and out of consciousness.

15

Dr. Russ Morton, a doctor with expertise in blood diseases, was called to assume Nancy's care. When, doctor-to-doctor, I asked him for the straight scoop in regard to what we were facing, he looked at the floor before engaging my eyes.

"Dr. Winn, Nancy is about as sick as a person can be. I don't know if we will be able to get her into remission." He paused, momentarily looked out the window, and before reengaging, took a quick gasp-like breath that could be heard across the room. "If we can't achieve a remission, she won't last the week . . . I am so very sorry."

His definitive words were like the period at the end of the sentence. Final. No, they were worse. They were like the space after the period at the end of a sentence at the end of the paragraph at the end of the essay. Nothing more to add. Nothing more to say.

If you are a praying person, please add Nancy to your list. If not, please take a moment to visualize and remember a good time you had with her. Though she is physically weak, her spirit is strong as always. I know she will feel your love.

Sincerely,

Winnie

The Patient Who Stopped My Heart

May 31, 2:15 a.m.

Dear Family,

As I sit beside Nancy and watch her breathe from my almost comfortable hospital chair, I am actively trying to force positive thoughts into my being. I want to write something to balance yesterday's note I sent you, so sad and so negative. I've always been an optimistic person, but this day has taxed me as no day before. My mind game worked. And I can now describe my "eureka" moment.

Though I often want to take each of my five-year-old patients home with me, absolutely enjoy the challenge of attempting to influence my all-knowing teen patients, and have had my heart warmed multiple times by those senior patients who share their vast wisdom and memories, in my thirty-one years of providing health care, only two patient encounters have made my heart skip beats, caused my hands to get sweaty, and left my mouth feeling as though I had been in the desert for a full day without water.

In 1978, my first job as a newly licensed physician was providing primary care at a single-doctor clinic in Mammoth, Wyoming, just inside the northern border of Yellowstone National Park. I was a "single doctor" in two ways. First, I was the sole doctor at the clinic. Second, at the time, I was not married.

The work was exhilarating. Most of my patients were park visitors who came from all over this country and from the far corners of the rest of the world. Practicing medicine in a remote setting meant my head was often in a book. And as

17

if learning on the go wasn't enough of a challenge, I had several unusual duties that came with providing medical care in a national park—like accompanying the rangers on selected backcountry rescues when they thought having a doctor along might be beneficial.

On this particular afternoon late in August 1978, I assisted the rangers on just such a rescue. I was away from the clinic for about two and a half hours. During my absence, a sick thirty-year-old came to the clinic looking for medical care. My front office clerk, Amy, explained the unusual situation: "I'm sorry, Dr. Winn is on a backcountry rescue and we don't know when he'll be back. There is another walk-in clinic at Yellowstone Lake. If you don't want to wait, you should go there."

"How far away is Yellowstone Lake?" the patient's accompanying friend, Patricia, inquired.

Amy replied, "With the normal summer traffic, oh, an hour and a half to two hours."

Patricia conferred with her sick friend who, I was later told, was already a little green around the edges and not too excited about getting back into a moving vehicle. "Let's wait a bit and hope," she told Amy.

Mobile phones were still a figment of some technologist's fervent imagination back then, but I did have access to a ranger radio. Right after the clinic patient decided to wait for my return, I radioed the ranger dispatcher to report we were fifteen minutes out and would be met by an ambulance to transport the backcountry patient to the nearest hospital, located two hours away in Bozeman, Montana. The dispatcher called Amy, who alerted the patient she had made the right decision.

When I arrived back at the clinic, transferred the wilderness patient with the broken leg to the ambulance, and went into the room to see my waiting patient, I was instantly captivated. My heart fluttered and my hands were moist. I had never experienced such a reaction before with a patient, or for that matter, a nonpatient. The woman sitting on the exam table had an inviting, gentle smile that paradoxically made me both nervous yet comfortable. Her pale-blue eyes seemed as vast as the sky. Her easy laugh, frequent despite her stomach discomfort, was infectious. And her inviting aura made my skin tingle and my mind wander. I shuffled through the encounter, talking as much about Yellowstone, her, and myself as I did about her medical complaint. The visit lasted over an hour, far more than the twenty minutes it should normally have taken for an examination.

After she left, my nurse asked if I was all right. My reply was simple. "I think I'm in love." I had rarely ever used those words. My nurse was speechless. So she brought me an aspirin.

(I thought I was the only one awake at this hour, but I just got tapped on the shoulder by Nancy's nurse's aide, who brought me volumes of paperwork to read and sign. I'd better go. I'll explain later why I am sharing my wandering thoughts from the middle of the night when sleep is so foreign.)

Fondly,

Winnie

A Life Turned Upside Down

May 31, 4:26 a.m.

Dear Family and Friends,

After my first communication, many of you attempted to call. I apologize for not answering, but I purposely turned off my mobile phone because I remain a wreck, unable to finish a sentence without a box of Kleenex.

Numerous times over the years, I've heard the statement, "My life was turned upside down." I now empathize, fully understanding those words. In the blink of an eye, every facet of my existence has changed. I am trying to sort out what to do with my kids, my medical practice, and most importantly, my beloved wife.

As a doctor, I am searching for a solution where there may be none. As Nancy's husband, I want to share her pain and suffering or lie in her place. I have felt helpless, if not hopeless. But finally, I realized there was something I could do. As Nancy's best friend, I can connect her to her wide array of supporters. In the last few hours, I've formulated a plan.

Since talking is difficult for me, I will do my best to keep you updated with periodic messages. My letters may be interrupted, as the last one was when the nurse's aide arrived in Nancy's room. They may be disjointed due to the tiredness of my mind and body. More likely than not, they may be written in the middle of the night. There may be several in one day or none for several days. But I pledge to keep you connected to Nancy as best I can.

That said, there are a few more thoughts:

1. Feel free to ask me questions. None are too stupid. As a doctor, I will try to explain what is going on medically. For

those of you with lots of medical knowledge, I apologize in advance if I oversimplify. For those of you to whom I don't explain well enough, just ask me again.

2. When I write, I will try to present a short italicized summary at the end of each note. Please feel free to skip to my "summation" if you are in a hurry. Though I may include a story from the past (as with my last letter) or describe current events at the time I am experiencing them, reading my sometimes-random reflections is in no way required or expected.

3. My last request I will only say a *single* time. And I will put it in CAPS because it is so important to me. If you only want the brief overview, then only read the italicized summary.

HOWEVER, IF YOU WANT TO OPT OUT OF MY UPDATES, FEEL FREE TO RESPOND WITH "TAKE ME OFF THE LIST." I UNDERSTAND COMPLETELY IF YOU DON'T WANT TO READ MY CONTEMPLATIONS. YOU WON'T HURT MY FEELINGS IF YOU OPT OUT. WE WILL ALWAYS BE FRIENDS.

My very best,

Winnie

Crazy in Love

May 31, 6:08 a.m.

Dear Family and Friends,

Though my legs ache with tiredness and my face has the numb and tingly feeling I often experience just before drifting off to sleep, ten minutes of no movement in my hospital chair does not turn my mind's lights out. After a little ice-cold water from the hallway water fountain awakens first my lips and thereafter my brain, I have decided to finish the story about the second time a patient elicited strong emotional feelings.

The second time is right now. The patient is the one who lies beside me, fighting for her life. Now more than ever, I realize the depth of my feelings for Nancy. Even after twenty-seven years, looking at her in the early morning light makes me excited and completely (and fully) alive. I can hardly wait for her eyes to open so I can hold her hand and place a kiss on her lips. It feels just as it did when we had our very first date.

If you hadn't already guessed, our first date was the night after Nancy's visit to the clinic in Yellowstone National Park when she and her friend, Patricia, decided to see if I would return promptly from my backcountry rescue mission. It now seems like fate that she waited rather than going elsewhere. If she had left the clinic, our paths would have never crossed.

After a long-distance romance that brought us together a mere twelve days over the next six months (because she lived far away in the city of Boston), Nancy and I got married. My friends thought I was crazy. (They were right. I was crazy about my gentle soul mate. And I still am.)

Summary: Nancy's illness has certainly led to a reaffirmation of my feelings for her. My love for Nancy is unwavering, as is my resolve to help her triumph in this battle.

Thanks,

Winnie

A Rock in the Face of a Storm

June 1, 11:13 a.m.

Dear Family and Friends,

A lot has happened in the past day. Nancy has received multiple transfusions—red blood cells to correct her anemia, platelets that contain the clotting factors to help stop the nosebleeds and bruising, and fresh frozen plasma that contains the blood products she was sorely missing. In addition, she received several liters of IV fluid because she was so dehydrated. At least temporarily, Nancy is feeling considerably better. The doctors and nurses simply shake their heads in disbelief when Nancy tells them, "Yes, I did work the whole day before my admission," and "Yes, I drove myself from the airport to the emergency room when I was finished working."

As I write, Nancy is peacefully snoozing in a cozy hospital bed. Sitting in a brown fake-leather hospital chair next to her, I am stroking the back of a delicate hand while avoiding the attached IV for the antibiotics and medicines she is receiving. Nancy has a clear plastic tube attached to her nose to administer oxygen, and there are wires extending from her chest, legs, and arms to three different monitors checking many of her bodily functions. Intermittently, one of the monitors will make a loud, irritating beeping sound indicating that Nancy is not breathing fast enough or that her heart has missed a beat. Each time one of the alarms sounds, my heart skips several beats even though I know that the alerts rarely reflect a serious problem. Nancy does not awaken for the alarms.

It is so different for me to be holding a patient's hand to give comfort rather than to feel a pulse, inspect a rash, or examine some form of irregularity. I try to ignore the monitors, the bedside chart numbers, and the conversations between the many nurses, lab technicians, X-ray specialists, and doctors who constantly enter our room unannounced to check on Nancy's status. My forehead sweats and I swallow my words so that I don't offer an observation or give advice. When one of Nancy's nurses asked the respiratory therapist a question this morning, I almost raised my hand like a middle school student. I am clearly out of my element.

Critically, sitting in this room is not about me. I focus on Nancy and not only stroke the back of her hand but hold it lightly between both of mine. I am pleased that her hand is no longer hot to my touch. For much of the day yesterday, I ran cold water over my own hands before holding Nancy's. She smiled once between naps and said, "You really feel good, Winnie." Despite her eyes closing before I could reply, those were the best words I heard the entire day.

I silently wonder as I watch her sleep, "What are you thinking, Nancy?" Though she looks peaceful, I worry about the fevers, the subsequent body aches, and the weakness she must feel. I lament, "What is it like to know you are facing terrible, terrible odds?" When I adjust Nancy's head on the pillow in hope of making her more comfortable, she often doesn't even awaken. A singular question lingers in my mind: "What more can I do?" It echoes time and time again. I am panicking.

But you know my Nancy well. There is a wisp of a smile on her lips, her face is serene, and her forehead is smooth. She is a rock in the face of our storm. Before drifting off today, she tapped my shoulder to motion me closer and then whispered as if telling me a secret, "Winnie, I'm worried about you. You need to eat something. You need fresh air. I'll be all right for the half hour it would take to leave the hospital. Didn't you notice? There are others who can watch over me. Isn't that why we're paying all these hospital workers who keep interrupting my TV shows?"

That's my Nancy. Only she could incite my first laugh in over two days.

Summary: The resident doctors just walked in the room. I will write more and summarize later today.

Hurriedly yours,

Winnie

The Importance of Kind Thoughts

June 1, 9:29 p.m.

Dear Family and Friends,

After reviewing what I sent you last time, I realize I did a horrible job. A recap is in order, especially since many of you have asked if it is appropriate to forward my correspondence to others—which it is. My "Friends and Family" recipient list is multiplying rapidly due to your efforts. Thanks for letting me know of others who have an interest in our journey. Also, thank you for the many kind thoughts you have sent to us. I read each message to Nancy, though only when she is asleep.

Why when she is asleep, you might wonder?

Two reasons.

First, Nancy's body is working so hard to fight the leukemia that she naps just about all the time. She falls asleep in the middle of our conversations, and she has not stayed awake for an entire TV show even if it is only a half hour in length.

Second, and more importantly, Nancy has never liked being the focus of attention. She doesn't quite approve yet of me writing you because she has difficulty with fuss from others. When she finally comes around, I will reread each and every one of your kind thoughts during an alert period. Like me, she will be overwhelmed. And she greatly appreciates your notes and prayers.

So, the recap:

As many of you are aware, about two months ago Nancy ended her furlough from American Airlines and returned to work as a flight attendant for ASA (Atlantic Southeast Airlines), a Delta Airlines affiliate. ASA has a Salt Lake City flight attendant base. For the first time in thirty-three years, Nancy didn't have to commute for her job to another city like she did with TWA before it was absorbed by American.

On day one of the three-day trip she was working before her hospitalization, she developed a nosebleed that started and then stopped spontaneously. However, on day two she experienced another bloody nose that didn't stop as easily. By day three of the trip, she had developed a rash, bruising, and a high fever. She went directly to the hospital from the airport when she arrived home two nights ago. She was feeling so sick that when she arrived at the emergency room, she left her car at the entrance because she didn't possess the strength to park and walk back from the lot.

The ER doctor took one look at Nancy, drew some blood, and immediately called a hematologist in to consult. Nancy's blood count was completely out of whack. Her white blood cell count, at 89,000, was more than ten times the normal count because immature cancer cells or "blasts" had been released "early" into her peripheral blood stream from her bone marrow. The white blood-making cells in the bone marrow where the cancer resides have squeezed out the parent cells that normally make platelets. Since platelets are integral in preventing bleeding, her lack of the platelets explains her nosebleeds and bruises. The same cancerous white cells in the bone marrow also impinge on her ability to produce red cells, leading to her anemia. Additionally, Nancy "presented," or arrived, with a high fever, raising the specter of a systemic infection.

Much to my astonishment and the surprise of the doctors, Nancy had absolutely no symptoms until the three days when she was on her overnight trip. Though I was shocked at how sick she appeared when I first saw her, I was completely taken aback when her hematologist, Dr. Morton, told me not only that he suspected that blood cancer leukemia was Nancy's diagnosis but also that her disease was at an advanced stage.

"How could she get so sick so quickly?"

"It happens," he replied simply.

Dr. Morton has indicated that we were extremely lucky to get her to the hospital before she developed a significant bleeding problem or contracted a serious infection in her brain or another vital organ. With her blood count so far off and her immunity so compromised, either of these events could have caused Nancy's immediate demise. But so far, so good. After exhaustive testing, Nancy has no signs of major bleeding and no evidence of serious infection.

In contrast to the good news about life-threatening infections and bleeding, Dr. Morton has expressed pessimism going forward. He has told me her very high blood count numbers and the rapidity of the illness reveal an aggressive disease. He says that fighting blood cancer is much more of a challenge for someone at fifty-seven, like Nancy, than it would be for someone who was twenty-seven. When he presented his summary to me, I nearly collapsed to the floor. He isn't certain he can get ahead of her disease. He isn't sure Nancy will survive a full week.

I don't know if it is possible for me to describe how his prognosis makes me feel. However, your many kind replies have buoyed my spirits more than I can yet express.

Summary: When Nancy arrived at the hospital three days ago, the doctor thought her death was imminent.

So much love,

Winnie

The Exorcising of Demons

June 1, 11:52 p.m.

Dear Family and Friends,

As the night advances, I've been reflecting on last evening. As you might imagine, it was a bad night. A *really, really* bad night. Demons have been everywhere in my head. I have desperately searched the Internet for answers to my many questions. "I'm a doctor after all," I tell myself. "Surely I can make sense of this situation. Surely I can find something to help Nancy out of this mess."

In reality, I don't want answers. I suspect anything I find will be unfavorable. Reading between my tears, I don't find anything to change my mood. Every article I discover confirms Dr. Morton's assessment of how progressive the illness is and what that potentially means.

Still I vow not give up hope. Or, at the very least, I will support Nancy during each step of whatever her journey will come to be. Earlier, after a normally inconsequential bump into the hospital bed gave her a nasty new bruise, I convinced Nancy to allow me to assist on bathroom trips. With IVs constantly running, those trips are frequent.

"I don't want to awaken you if you are sleeping," she initially told me. I pointed to the fresh bruise on her left thigh and gave her a look I hadn't used since the kids were teens. "All right," she replied to my unstated words and added, "You always seem to be awake anyway." Nancy now allows me to rub her sore back and fetch her chocolate ice cream. By the end of last night, she understood. "You're not going anywhere, are you?" "No, I'm not," I replied as tears yet once again filled my eyes.

Our new temporary home has one small window, approximately two feet square. From Nancy's bed and the chair where I sit and sleep, the east-facing view provides a mostly unobstructed look at the Wasatch Mountains. The entire evening last night, I looked forward to seeing the snow-covered horizon if only to be comforted by knowing that our real home is somewhere amid the foothills. When the dark of night transitioned to the light of dawn, slate-gray clouds initially obscured the distant peaks. It was just another disappointment to add to a growing list.

However, right before the doctors arrived on their morning rounds today, the clouds disappeared. Our window was filled with mountaintops jutting into a sky bright with sunshine. When the doctors arrived, they brought even brighter news.

Nancy's diagnosis has been confirmed. She is fighting acute myeloid leukemia, or AML for short. This particular leukemia has six subgroups, and Dr. Morton explained that Nancy has the rare one called M3. Of the six, M3 has the best prognosis. Statistically, M3 AML has an approximately 70% cure rate. Several of the other subgroups have cure rates of less than 2%, which is what I had read about before I forced myself to another task. And as I held my breath, Dr. Morton grabbed my hand and looked me straight in the eyes: "Winnie, this changes everything. We should be able to get Nancy into remission even though her blood count is so seriously altered." We shook hands vigorously.

So in less than forty-eight hours, Nancy has a solid diagnosis. And after a single five-minute conversation, my spirits jumped to above the mountains outside our tiny window. Even the sterile and stale hospital room air suddenly smelled fresher. The light in the room seemed brighter. I took a bite of Nancy's unfinished hospital "everything" bagel, and it actually tasted like a gourmet bagel that exploded my taste buds with a multitude of flavors.

I savored the moment and let Dr. Morton's words pervade and wash over my being.

Nancy should make it through this week!

It is miraculous how quickly our fate has changed.

When Nancy was first admitted, it was Memorial Day weekend. Initially, I worried nothing would happen until Tuesday and that I might have to take a nurse hostage to get a hematologist to come see her. I even fantasized picketing the hospital cafeteria to get her initial blood tests done.

But now, instead of being frustrated and angry, I am celebrating this holiday weekend. As I write, our medical team not only has secured the diagnosis but is now hanging the IV fluid containing Nancy's first chemotherapy treatment.

Our journey has begun.

We are now ready to tackle the day-to-day tasks. We have to think about nutrition, exercise, and the routine tests that Nancy will have pretty much every day. She does not need the painful procedure called a bone marrow extraction, since her AML diagnosis was so obvious. We are happy with that news since it means one less needle. Nancy faces many, many prods and sticks in the coming days and weeks. Presently, she has three separate IVs going into her body. When the chemotherapy side effects kick in, she may not be able to eat, which might mean more procedures and tubes. Still, Nancy's smile is fully back. And mine is slowly beginning to emerge again.

OK. You are current on Nancy's status. If my explanation doesn't make sense, it might be because I am on the last of my adrenaline having been up continuously over the last several days. Even toothpicks can't keep my eyes open, and I am probably rambling with nonsense.

Feel free to send questions so I can address them.

We're in this for the long haul, and both of us really appreciate your support. I have no doubt that if anyone can beat this thing, it is my Nancy.

P.S. Nancy is not allowed to receive flowers due to the fragility of her immune system and the resulting worry about infection. Originally, my plan was to fill her room with the largest array of colors and varieties in Utah. I was going to set aside time for a mountain bike ride in quest of buckets of spring wild flowers, which I planned to supplement with the best blossoms and plants the local florist had on hand. I also assumed Nancy might receive a few flowers from some of you. But, unfortunately, no flowers for now.

However, if you'd like to send a card, Nancy's address for at least the next several weeks is: LDS Hospital, Room 842 East, 8th and C Street, Salt Lake City, Utah 84143.

Summary: Nancy is a different person than I wrote about yesterday. Her spirits are high. She is feeling stronger and ready to fight the good fight. Most importantly, her prognosis has changed. She still has a serious, life-threatening illness. But now there is hope.

Love to you all,

Winnie

A Sack Full of Stones

June 2, 8:24 p.m.

Dear Family and Friends,

I am overwhelmed with the outpouring of love that you've sent Nancy and our family. I don't know if I could have survived these past few days without such unconditional support. Many of you have asked about our two children, Jaret and Jayna. Where are they? How are they coping? I will save Jaret for a future note, but tonight is a suitable occasion to address Jayna.

Two weeks ago today, Jayna called from Cusco, Peru, where she has just completed her Junior Year Abroad coursework toward a Latin American Studies degree from Vassar College. Her voice was full of excitement.

"I'm finished, Dadder. I learned so much."

I can forever visualize my daughter's always expressive face. Twinkling blue eyes above a warm, tooth-filled, disarming smile. A childlike excitement in the way her eyebrows lift as she speaks. A flip of her head to position her darkish-blonde bangs back across her forehead. She's inherited so much from Nancy.

"What would you think of me staying awhile? I kind of met a guy I like . . ."

I hoped Jayna couldn't hear what to me was a very loud swallow. I wanted to scream, "No way, Jayna! You are my little girl, and I don't want you to be with any guy. South America is too far away from Utah. We were only able to visit you once last year, and it nearly killed your mother and me."

Though those thoughts rattled in my head while I weighed an answer, I couldn't ignore the fact that Jayna is, put simply, a fine young woman. She was valedictorian in high school. She is idealistic and wants to save the world. She is genuinely kind, warm, and loving.

To be fair, at times she was a challenge as a kid, but she was mischievous rather than troublesome. And yes, she loves to argue with me and point out when I am wrong or inconsistent—or both. But Jayna is so vibrant and full of life that she can melt me on the spot with a grab of my hand, a kiss on my cheek, or the "look" that reinforces what she often verbalizes.

"I do remember what you've taught me, Dadder. Friends and family are the most important things in life. And yes, Dadder. You are family."

"Well, I guess staying a little longer would be OK," I responded trying to mask my reluctance. "Do you need anything?"

"No, Dadder, I've already got a job. I'll be home in a month."

Did I mention that Jayna is independent and adventuresome?

"I do miss you both a lot. Thank goodness for mobile phones and the Internet."

It was therefore with a considerable weight on my shoulder that felt like a full sack of stones that I finally picked up the phone this morning to inform Jayna about her mother's illness.

Nancy, of course, urged me not to call.

"I really don't want to ruin Jayna's special time in a faraway country. She is too young to have to deal with something like this."

Jayna and Nancy are as close as any mother and daughter. And I knew that Jayna would want to hear from me as strongly as Nancy didn't want her to hear at all.

Over the years, due to caring for visiting tourists as part of my day job, I've gained experience in making difficult calls to faraway family members. But experience doesn't help when calling your own faraway daughter. As I dialed the long international number, I had to concentrate on not spilling over with emotion.

"Jayna, it's Dad."

"Dadder, is something wrong?"

So much for my charade. Nancy often teases me about being transparent.

After trying to disguise my audible deep breath by momentarily putting my hand over the phone, I answered, "Yes, Jayna, there is . . . Mom is sick."

Now it was Jayna's voice that sounded distressed. She pleaded, "Sick? How sick, Dad?"

"Real sick. She has the blood cancer called acute myeloid leukemia."

There was an uncomfortable delay not due to the connection. "Cancer? Mom has cancer? Do I need to come home?"

"Yes." I had hoped to elaborate but could not find any words.

Jayna replied softly, "Dadder, I'll make arrangements. I'll call you back in a little while with details."

"Thanks, Jayna."

"Dadder? Tell Mom I love her. And that I'll be there soon."

Jayna called me back within the hour. She had already packed her things, said good-bye to her friends, and made a reservation to be on the next plane to Utah that had space, leaving the next night and arriving (with connections and such) the following day.

She ended our call with, "We can do this, Dadder. I'm ready." There had been no second thoughts about coming and no doubts about her role.

How many twenty-two-year-olds are willing to put their lives on hold instantaneously? (I know at least one.)

When Jayna called initially, Nancy had been asleep. When she awakened about an hour later, I told her the news. She scrunched her eyebrows toward her nose, thrust her lower lip forward, and waved her index finger at me. The feigned anger morphed into the largest smile I have ever seen on my bride's face. Shortly thereafter, tears were streaming down Nancy's cheeks. It was the first time she had cried (unlike me).

"Tomorrow?" she asked, not needing an answer. I hugged Nancy tightly. Surprisingly, though Nancy has been weakened by her ordeal, her return hug rivaled mine in strength.

Lastly, tonight before I tucked Nancy between the starchy white hospital sheets and under the lime-green hospital blanket, she looked at me with those big sky-blue eyes of hers, and with a new bounce in her voice, she directed, "Can you add . . ." and gave me three new names to put on my update list.

I guess I'll have a lot of catch-up reading to do so that Nancy will know how thoughtful all of you have been.

We've come a long, long way.

On the other hand, Nancy is still adjusting to hospital life.

Most of you can probably imagine her telling the nurse or aide that he or she doesn't need to "make an extra trip" and me interrupting with, "Thank you. If you would bring that cold washcloth for Nancy's forehead it would be wonderful!"

I have such an incredible soul mate. Between naps this afternoon, she even helped Jaret with the final paper for his spring semester at Westminster College.

Summary: Jayna will arrive home from Peru the day after tomorrow to be with her mom and support her dad. None too soon.

Much love,

Winnie

The Hospital Roller Coaster

June 3, 1:37 p.m.

Dear Friends and Family,

How can a single day have such extremes?

Leukemia—the name on the side of our new personal roller coaster.

Let me explain.

This morning, I awakened feeling positive and upbeat. Jayna is set to board a plane this evening. Nancy has been cleared to begin a new drug specific to her AML subtype, M3. Our nurse even brought me my very own breakfast tray from a patient who had gone for surgery, thereby saving a trip to the cafeteria. Bright and cheery, Nancy commanded me to concentrate on my "other" patients. "Go to work," she declared, pointing to the large, round clock on the wall opposite her bed, "It's time . . ." I swallowed the last bite of French toast and raced to the parking lot.

As I drove up the mountain to Park City from Salt Lake City where I spent the night in my now familiar chair, it almost felt like a normal day. Within a half hour, I had treated one of my favorite patients, seven-year-old Johnny Hernandez, for strep throat and followed that with putting stitches into the arm of one of Jayna's classmates, Amanda Lester. Unlike when sitting in Nancy's hospital room, I felt the power of providing care rather than witnessing it. I walked taller than I have in days.

In an instant, however, *everything has changed.*

As prearranged, Nancy's nurse called my mobile phone with the morning progress report just as I had requested. Her voice was flat. "Things are not so good here, Winnie. You better come right away." I didn't ask for nor want details.

37

My partners have already made their support clear. After the emergency meeting they held the day I told them about Nancy's illness, I received a unanimous message relayed by Joe Ferriter, our CEO: "Work as much or as little as is best for your family, Winnie. We will cover you."

As a result, with no hesitation, I told my medical assistant, Mindy, I was leaving, threw my stethoscope in my desk drawer, and sprinted for the exit seconds after I hung up with Nancy's nurse. I was lucky there were no patrol officers on the highway to Salt Lake City. Not a single car passed me while speeding down the mountain on Interstate 80.

Twenty-five minutes after exiting the clinic, I was back in my now accustomed chair next to Nancy's bed, hanging on every word uttered by her oncologist, Dr. Elizabeth Prystas.

"Most leukemics start off treatment pretty well, and at about two weeks, things get a little bit rough. However, with Nancy's M3 type of leukemia, things are going to get tough right away. I know it's distressing seeing Nancy struggle, but it's not uncommon for this to happen."

I glanced at Nancy beside me on the bed. Her face was mostly obscured by the oxygen mask covering it, delivering 15 liters (or 45%) of inspired oxygen. I wished I didn't know that 15 liters was a very high concentration of oxygen for any patient to receive. Despite the oxygen, Nancy was working hard just to breathe. Each of her breaths was rapid and labored. Through the mask, I could see that her face was puffy, as were the tissues surrounding her eyes. Worse yet, her futile attempt to give Dr. Prystas a brief smile was familiar to me.

Pain.

My stomach was tied in knots. For most of the conversation, Nancy appeared far away. Dr. Prystas witnessed what I saw as well. She stopped trying to include Nancy in our discussion. When Nancy's eyes closed, Dr. Prystas motioned for me to join her in the hallway. I squeezed Nancy's hand and blew her a kiss as I left the room. Nancy's eyes remained shut. She didn't squeeze back.

Dr. Prystas closed the door and continued: "Nancy started a new chemotherapy medicine, ATRA, this morning. Though it's very specific in fighting her type of leukemia, it sometimes causes breathing problems. However, we still have to consider other possibilities. She could have a lung infection. Or she could be bleeding into her lungs from her low platelets. If Nancy gets worse, we'll put her in the intensive care unit. As I'm sure you noticed, we're already supplementing her oxygen at the highest level. If it's not enough or she tires from her increased breathing effort, she may need respiratory support. We've asked a pulmonologist to help us."

I could feel my face flush and my legs weaken. Nancy might be transferred to the ICU? She might need a respirator? A lung specialist will see her? As I connected the dots, I leaned against the wall, in need of support. The unthinkable stared me in the face.

Could Nancy die after a single day of the new treatment?

What happened to the 70% cure rate?

All I could mumble to Dr. Prystas was, "Thanks for keeping me informed."

Dr. Prystas momentarily put her hand on my shoulder, nodded her respectful condolence, and turned away and headed down the hall.

How could things have gone so wrong, so rapidly?

Last night Nancy looked almost normal. We talked and laughed (and I cried when she fell asleep). She slept the entire night. She shooed me away to work.

But now?

Nancy was far away. And struggling. I pulled my chair close to her bed and put her hand between both of mine. Again. My mind raced.

Will Jayna get home from Peru in time?

Why did I think I could go to work today?

And the one question that has become my daily personal balancing act: Is it time to call Nancy's mother, sister, and brother in Georgia again?

Summary: Things are not going well right now.

Love,

Winnie

The Power of Determination
June 3, 10:30 p.m.

Dear Friends and Family,

When I wrote earlier today, I felt like the world was ending. It was so incredibly hard to see the love of my life fight for each and every breath. My hands felt like twenty-pound weights; I couldn't even open my computer, let alone type. I silently prepared for the worst.

Seconds seemed like minutes. Minutes seemed like hours. Nurses and respiratory therapy technicians were my constant companions. Nancy had two sets of X-rays done right in our room because she was too sick to go to the radiology suite. The pulmonologist, the lung specialist, came and went and came again.

His report?

"All of her tests are inconclusive so far, Dr. Winn. If need be, we will do a lung biopsy. In the meantime, if she worsens, we'll need to intervene. I've started her on steroids. They sometimes help in these cases."

He didn't elaborate any more than this, knowing I knew what he meant. He didn't mention that if Nancy had a lung infection, steroids could make her much worse.

Though Nancy squeezed my hand a few times, she mostly continued to be far away. I did notice, however, a different look on her face even though it was swollen.

Determination.

The look on her face transported me back in time to twenty-five years ago. Nancy was pregnant with Jaret. Like many first-time expectant moms, Nancy did everything right: no medicines, no alcohol, exercise, classes about delivery, and books about child development. We looked forward to a "perfect" birth. After talking to her friends who had already experienced labor, reading about different birth methods, and discussing all of the options with my medical partner, Tom Schwenk, who was slated to deliver her, Nancy announced her decision. "I want to go natural, Tom."

Nancy jogged two miles every morning until the day her water broke. She was physically and mentally prepared for our first child. Her bag had been packed for weeks. As we pulled out of the driveway on the way to the hospital, she declared, "O . . . K," and gave me a thumbs up. I was frightened. She was not. When we were halfway down the mountain and I glanced at her beside me, I saw "the look" for the first time. I was both reassured and excited.

Childbirth can be fickle. Though Nancy grabbed my hand often and smiled the best she could through her increasingly frequent pains, the labor dragged on and on and on. In fact, she progressed so slowly that I once fell asleep while leaning against the wall. When I awoke minutes later, Nancy's visage remained unchanged. She was doing far better than me.

Determination.

Two full nurse shifts later, our original nurse from the previous day returned. She was shocked that we were still there. "I didn't expect to see you. How's it going?"

I would have answered "not well." Nancy's expression reported differently.

Before Nancy could verbalize, Tom entered our room, reviewed her chart, and examined Nancy. His assessment was blunt: "Nancy, it has been a full twenty-six hours of labor. If you won't let me give you medicine, you could end up with a C-section. That would not be best for you or the baby."

Thirty minutes later, after an epidural helped relax Nancy, our son Jaret entered the world. And when he looked at his tired but happy mother, I am sure he saw the last vestiges of the same look that I see on Nancy's face today. Like then, I know that whatever the outcome, Nancy is giving it her all.

Determination.

As the daylight shining through our window began to fade, so did Nancy's oxygen needs. The nurses began to smile on their frequent visits. So did Nancy. Her face regained its radiance and gradually lost its swelling. Within three hours, her breathing returned to normal. Within four hours, the oxygen mask was gone.

A miracle?

I have learned that in some patients, the drug ATRA causes breathing problems that are transient and responsive to steroids. The miracle is that Nancy is a member of this group. We survived a serious scare, and as the day has progressed to night, the sparkle has returned to those beautiful sky-blue eyes. Needless to say, I have ascended from the depths of fear and depression to near ecstasy in the course of twelve hours.

Summary: Nancy is feeling and looking good again.

Full of love for all those
around me including you,

Winnie

Hepburn and Tracy

June 4, 11:51 p.m.

Dear Friends and Family,

With Nancy working as a flight attendant for over thirty years, I have often joked that I could drive to the airport blindfolded.

In our early married years before the 9/11 tragedy, I would wait for her at the gate whenever possible. It was so romantic to have her stroll down the jetway and into my arms. It felt like we were in a Katherine Hepburn and Spencer Tracy movie. Our passionate hugs were soon replaced by those with Jaret and Jayna, who would jump up and down as Nancy deplaned, screaming "Mommy, Mommy!" before leaping into her outstretched arms.

Even after access to the gate became a distant memory, it was still special to pick up Nancy after she had been working for several days in far-off cities. It is safe to say that airports in general, and Salt Lake City International Airport in particular, have always been an integral part of our family's makeup. However, as I drove to the airport today, I could not recall ever feeling more nervous anticipation.

When Jayna emerged from the door outside the baggage claim area, time stood still. Even though it had only been two months since I had last seen her, in the few seconds I had to observe her from afar before she met my eyes, waved, and sprinted to our car, she appeared years older and more mature. Anyone who saw us must have wondered what was going on. We hugged and clung to each other not speaking a word, but both of us had tears flowing down our faces not in single drops

43

but rather in rivers, our bottled up emotions finally having a safe outlet. The security guard approached to tell me to move my car, but seeing Jayna's face first and then catching my glance, waved his hand in a "never-mind" gesture.

After several minutes of clinging tightly to one another, Jayna spoke, "Can we go the hospital?"

When we entered the room, Nancy was snoring. Jayna looked at me and gave me a "thumbs up" gesture as if to say, "She doesn't look so bad." I was so very glad she hadn't seen her mom twenty-four hours earlier.

Before I could make up my mind whether or not I should awaken her, Nancy opened her eyes, raised her eyebrows, and extended her arms. Jayna was soon lying beside her mom, her head resting on her mom's chest. Nancy's nurse entered the room, looked at the scene, handed me a pill to give Nancy later, and left quickly.

Jayna simply lit up the room for both Nancy and me.

The rest of the evening was joyous. The chatter was non-stop, like preteens at a slumber party. Nancy stayed up a full two hours catching up on Jayna's exploits even though she was tired from the day's ordeal. Jayna kissed her mom's cheek and after noticing her mother's difficulty in keeping her eyes open said, "Mom, you're tired. Close your eyes. I will be here when you wake up." Seconds later, Nancy's body made a now familiar jerk that told me she was already in a deep slumber.

Summary: A small amount of order has returned to our world. Our family is reunited once again; Jayna arrived home this afternoon.

The very best,

Winnie

Random Thoughts in a Dark Room

June 5, 2:00 a.m.

Dear Friends and Family,

When Nancy's nurse entered the room to check vital signs late tonight, I was startled, momentarily not sure where I was. Wide-awake, I gathered my bearings and decided there was no better time to write you once again than in the quiet darkness. My open computer shed enough light to illuminate a new piece of furniture in our "temporary" home. Our very own rollaway bed. Fast asleep beneath her very own lime-green hospital blanket was Jayna, exhausted from the long journey and the day's events. The bed's arrival was timely not just because our "slumber party" had the two of us spending the night with Nancy. Just before she'd drifted off to dreamland, Jayna and I formulated a new plan. She and I will alternate spending the night so that Nancy will *never* be alone. I look forward to the rollaway even though, at this point, I am almost used to "my" chair.

I do want to put the day in perspective. It ended magnificently.

Unlike the morning and early afternoon, the day before yesterday when Nancy looked horrible and in the evening when she had improved but was drained from the ordeal, when Jayna arrived yesterday, her mom both felt and looked good. No doubt, Jayna was a major contributor. Her presence alone has raised Nancy's spirits multiple octaves. My girls' frequent laughter fills the room and is music to my ears. A dab of Passion Flower perfume to her mother's neck, one of many gifts that appeared from Jayna's suitcase, left the rest of the evening without the sterile hospital smell to which I'd nearly become accustomed.

I savored the evening, knowing that tomorrow Nancy restarts the ATRA pills that cause such dramatic side effects. I am told that any negative consequences are usually less intense the second time around, and hopefully that will be the case. However, these dramatic side effects clearly demonstrate that each step in our journey is a crapshoot.

We can't get too high.

We can't get too low.

Our race is a marathon, not a sprint.

Things can quickly turn bad.

And just as quickly get better.

Earlier I forgot to report some promising details. In just seven days, many of Nancy's lab abnormalities are improving. Even her white blood count, previously made up largely of the "bad guy" cancer cells, has dropped from 89,000 to 13,000. We'd like the number to be about 8,000, with those cells being normal ones rather than leukemic white cells.

Today's numbers demonstrate that the chemotherapy meds are definitely doing their job. If only we are able to maintain the balance between side effects and effectiveness.

Our hopes are high.

There were several other highlights today, too.

We've received many presents for Nancy's room. Thanks. I still wish I could fill every nook and cranny with flowers, but "oh well." I do want to acknowledge a very clever gift, sent not to us but instead to the hospital staff. One of our special friends, Debbi Fields (of Mrs. Fields Cookies), sent box after box of cookies, cakes, and other delicious snacks. Large containers of coffee and juice arrived as well. A long folding table was set up in the hall next to the nurse's station to accommodate the sheer volume of treats. The accompanying card read, "Please take good care of my dear friend, Nancy."

Staff and hospital visitors congregated nearby not only to eat the many treats but also to breathe in the strong, fresh aromas. The coffee was hot and the cookies still warm. Our already excellent care is now delivered with satisfied smiles reflecting full bellies.

Mmmm.

Thanks, Debbi; you are a dear, dear friend.

Jayna also has brought home various good luck charms from Peru that she has used to add pizzazz to the dull, metal IV pole standing guard over Nancy's bed. A Peruvian native medicine doctor, called a "shaman," blessed the most striking one, composed of two multicolored feathers attached to a crystal star that captures and reflects light like a rainbow.

When Nancy fell asleep near midnight, Jayna and I quietly decorated the rest of the room with hanging plastic flowers and balloons from the gift shop that now highlight your many gifts, cards, and pictures. They can be viewed in every direction from Nancy's bed, and she stated it best before she fell asleep, "I am surrounded by so much love."

Meanwhile, Jayna whispered to me, "We need to make this room 'home,' Dadder," In the quiet moments, she composed a long list of the other things she wants to purchase. In hindsight, I guess I've been too focused on machines, lab results, and Nancy to notice how stark and dreary the hospital room appears—that is, before Jayna. As I look at Jayna sleeping on the rollaway bed, the tears always seem to well up.

Finally, I want to report about our first nonfamily visitor.

Around dinnertime, there was a knock on our door. When I opened it, Anne Evers (the wife of my partner Bob Evers) was standing just to the side so as not to be in Nancy's view. "I know Nancy is not having visitors yet," she said softly, "but I wondered if you can take a field trip with me." (Anne works in the special hematology lab that follows blood diseases like AML.) Minutes later, we were in the hospital basement, winding through a maze of tunnels before arriving at Anne's lab.

"Look," she said as she adjusted the microscope for me. "Those big ones are Nancy's leukemic cells." I adjusted the focus on Anne's microscope to clearly view the "bad guy" cells. Gazing at Nancy's foe elicited a rush of passion different from the multitude of emotions that cycles daily through my being.

The strong new feeling?

Anger.

Anne, reading my face, grabbed my hand: "It's going to be all right, Winnie. Now you've seen the enemy."

We both laughed a bit nervously. After another extended look, the anger dissipated as quickly as it had appeared. Without embarrassment, I declared out loud to the microscopic cells I had just viewed, "You're toast!"

Crazy, huh? Anne was tickled and repeated my assessment.

One last detail I nearly forgot. After sitting at the foot of Nancy's bed, watching and sending positive energy in her direction for many hours yesterday afternoon, I discovered something new about my bride. Nancy has elegant ankles. Sleek, strong lines. A few bruises from the decreased platelets and clotting factors, but her veins don't stick out like they do on my ankles. The bumps on either side protrude gently, again in contrast to many I've examined over the years.

Nancy's ankles are simply quite lovely. I held them for several hours today.

Even after twenty-seven years, I am learning new things about Nancy. What isn't new is her dignity and grace in the face of adversity and her worry about bothering all of you. Though she isn't completely sold on me writing you yet, she does send you her best and looks forward to future connections.

I will try to update you again in several days.

By then, I may even have a better sense of how we're doing.

Summary: Today ended with Nancy feeling better and some positive lab results. We are ready for tomorrow.

My very best,

Winnie

A Week Is a Very Long Time

June 6, 5:22 a.m.

Dear Friends and Family,

Last night was a special anniversary. (No, not of our marriage. I look forward to that too, many months away.) Yesterday marked the end of the first full week in our new (hospital room) home. I had a good cry in the bathroom down the hall when I realized the significance.

One week ago yesterday, Nancy's doctor told me she might not be with us for this long. I decided not to remind Nancy or Jayna and instead toasted the smiling yet very wet face in the mirror with a paper cup full of cold, fresh water. Funny, the tap water tasted at least as good as wine. But the best anniversary present came from the sleep spirits.

As seems to be my habit, I awakened in time to view the sun jump atop the majestic Wasatch Mountains through our east-facing window. I found, somewhat surprisingly, that watching the sun's energy rouse the Salt Lake Valley was mesmerizing. Tall, glass-filled office buildings reflected a rainbow of color from the sun's initial rays. The first delivery trucks darted quickly down otherwise empty streets. The sudden rise in temperature allowed four black-tailed hawks to take advantage of the morning updraft and glide gracefully through space.

And the best part of my view was not outside the room—but rather just to my immediate left. Nancy was still peacefully sleeping, having had her longest slumber of the week, a full seven and a half hours. She only stirred to swallow her midnight pills, to provide an arm for her 5 a.m. blood draw, and to lend an ear for a temperature determination during her vital

49

signs checks that are being done every four hours. It was her best night yet. In fact, for most of the night, Nancy slept deeply enough to snore. (Don't tell her I told you.)

During her 11 p.m. blood draw, just before kissing my cheek goodnight, she described a dream from the previous evening: "It was really weird, Winnie. I was both the nurse and the patient. I took my own temperature, dispensed pills to myself from a bottle the size of a gallon of milk, and went to the hospital kitchen and served myself a plate overflowing with blueberry pancakes stacked at least six inches high. I even started my own IV. It didn't hurt."

I chuckled along with Nancy at her retelling, but I am excited and happy—even subconsciously Nancy is becoming part of her treatment. She certainly does all of the other necessary things to help herself get better. Several times a day, she walks the halls, IV in tow and mask on her face.

Last night, out of the blue, Nancy said, "Why don't we see if the TV works?"

We watched an entire NBA playoff game between my team and the Golden State Warriors. By halftime, I was so relaxed that I could reflect without worry that today Nancy restarted her chemotherapy meds and there have been no untoward effects. That same drug nearly put her on a respirator seventy-two hours ago. This time, it was totally innocuous.

Myself, I probably slept five hours—my best hospital sleep as well. (In the comfort category, the rollaway is a quantum leap from the chair.) For the first time since Nancy's diagnosis, I am actually feeling well rested because every other night I am home in Woodland in a real bed, secure with the knowledge that Nancy is in very capable hands—Jayna's.

Jayna. Though she immediately dropped everything in Peru and traveled twenty-six hours straight to be at her mom's side, Jayna strolled into the hospital and has not missed a beat.

Well, maybe an occasional beat. When Jayna is tired, she'll burst into Spanish before she notices the dim-witted look on my face signifying I have no clue what she has just said.

I am elated to have her back.

Jayna is like her mom. She has an incredible presence and similarly gutsy determination. She single-handedly helped wean Nancy off oxygen yesterday by challenging her to excel during a breathing exercise that entailed sucking air out of a machine. Unfortunately, all hospitals are staffed differently than when I was a resident, so minor nursing care like Nancy's breathing exercise is left to the family. Jayna is up to the task. Nancy nicknamed Jayna "the slave driver," a badge Jayna wears proudly. In comparison, I would probably be labeled "old softy."

Jayna's effect on me has been equally dramatic. With our tag teaming at the hospital, I can see patients at the clinic knowing Nancy is not alone; ride my mountain bike almost every day with Chuck or Kathleen, who want me to stay healthy so I can help Nancy recover; and do mundane house stuff like making sure Nancy's many houseplants don't weaken and wither.

When I search for silver linings to the terrible hand we've been dealt, one particular example screams out.

Parents don't routinely watch their children grow, mature, and demonstrate their value systems. In our case, Nancy's leukemia has provided a dramatic window into the woman our daughter has become as an adult. When Jayna called this morning to inquire about her mom's night and tell me she was on her way to the hospital to relieve me, she dropped a bombshell: "Dadder, I've decided. I won't be returning to Vassar this fall. I need to be with you and Mom."

My heart plunged and I had an acid-like taste so bad I needed two Tums tablets. Nancy and I want Jayna's senior year at Vassar to be the best. With a 3.87 GPA, she has mastered the academic challenges. A tremendous group of caring friends have been discovered. And she would have returned fresh from an entire year's adventure in Peru, full of perspective and wisdom to enjoy her last carefree college days. Nancy and I want her senior year in college to be the end of the educational rainbow.

And yet Jayna is poised to put her traditional college experience in the rearview mirror. "Jayna, that's three months away. No need to decide now," I meekly replied as we hung up.

I live my days in halves.

I work half the time in Park City treating a large number of patients, and the other half at the hospital worrying about a single patient. On my days off from the clinic, when I am in Woodland, everyday details replace patient care: paying bills, getting the garage door fixed, transferring the dirty dishes from the sink into the dishwasher. I haven't allowed myself to think about anything farther than two days into the future.

My daughter on the other hand?

She is already thinking months ahead.

When Jayna arrived at the hospital later in the day for her "shift," she finished our conversation: "Dadder, I mourned Vassar for two full days. I'm ready to move forward. I have an appointment tomorrow at the U. I might just finish college here in Utah."

As I looked into Jayna's sparkling blue eyes and basked in the warmth of her smile, I saw both peace and resolve.

She is so much like her mother.

My head was filled with the unspoken words from our good friend Joannie.

"Jayna was born wise."

Summary: I am trying not to exhale because we're savoring a "good time" period, in no small part due to Jayna.

Much love,

Winnie

A Mother's Son

June 7, 6:48 p.m.

Dear Friends and Family,

Many of you have inquired about Jaret. So I will dedicate this note to him. (I have been remiss in not including an update on him sooner, as he, like Jayna, is an important part of our team. There are so many puzzle pieces to keep on the board.)

Jaret (who we often call J) is now twenty-five years old.

As many of you know, Jaret is autistic, though fortunately he is very high functioning. His major disability is extreme shyness that makes it difficult for him in social interactions. When he talks, he rarely looks you in the eye. He also has weak fine motor strength that makes tasks like cutting his own finger- and toenails a personal challenge and the act of writing an adventure. (Thank goodness for computers, as his penmanship is as illegible as mine.)

Intellectually, he has great strengths in his areas of interest where he is almost an expert and creates his own world with each of the fields he enjoys. He performed well enough in high school and on the ACT test to be accepted at Westminster College in Salt Lake City, where he is living independently amid his junior year and carrying a 3.4 GPA.

As you could probably guess, much of his strength and success is a direct result of his mother's unwavering love, support, and advocacy. Her kind, gentle manner has always made him feel safe and secure, empowering him to push *his* envelope and reach *his* full potential. For example, many individuals with autism don't travel well because they need a strict routine to feel comfortable. Jaret, on the other hand, has grown up exploring various parts of the globe because it is part of his mother's world.

In the past, Jaret has been averse to all issues surrounding death. He abhors Halloween and costumes, closes his eyes when we pass graveyards in the car, and doesn't like to hear any of my medical stories the way Jayna does. So Jaret has been hit especially hard by Nancy's sickness.

"Could Mom die, Dad?" he asked the first night after I explained Nancy's disease.

A most difficult conversation followed. But like his sister, Jaret has risen to the occasion.

"I'll be okay, Dad. You help Mom." And without hesitation or complaint, Jaret regularly visits his mom in the hospital, a place that he previously avoided much like he does vegetables.

So Jaret is doing well. He is finishing this semester and, for the first time, without his mother's constant vigilance and assistance. Many of you have kindly offered help. Right now, it appears Jaret doesn't need it. In a single week, he has grown up years.

Summary: With his mother's illness, Jaret has been forced to be more independent than ever before. He has been up to the challenge. He is his mother's son.

All our love,

Winnie

The Red Assassin

June 7, 8:39 p.m.

Dear Friends and Family,

Nancy and Jayna spent much of the day shopping for hats on line.

Why?

Nancy just completed the last dose of one of her chemotherapy drugs, Idarubicin. Idarubicin's job is to attack bone marrow cells, but it affects other rapidly growing cells, like hair, as well. Though it often upsets the GI tract, it hasn't even made Nancy nauseated. My strong woman—a woman, nonetheless, whose hair is falling out in clumps. (I am afraid to share with you that very soon my bride will have less hair than me.)

Idarubicin is very ascetically impressive when administered because it is a bright red, almost fluorescent liquid. Anyone witnessing it trickle down the IV tubing and into Nancy's vein can't help but believe it must be powerful.

I think all IV meds should have color. But even if Idarubicin wasn't red, it truly is a potent medicine. I have therefore nicknamed it "The Assassin Drug" because it is meant to obliterate Nancy's entire bone marrow.

At the suggestion of our good friend Marion Wheaton (a nurse), each time Nancy gets it, I visualize miniature "Pac-Men" entering her bloodstream to eat up the "evil" white cells. As an alternative, Marion suggested thinking about little soldiers marching to battle, so I now ask Nancy to visualize an army parading into her vein. (She gives me that "Yes, dear" look.)

The Assassin Drug, full of "Pac-Men" or soldiers, has been busy.

Nancy's white blood count (WBC) is now a shadow of its former self, a mere four hundred. Not the 89,000 WBC it was on admission. Or the 4,000 WBC that would be on the low end of the normal WBC range of about 4,500–10,000.

FOUR HUNDRED!

This very low number is really good news, leukemia-wise. It means, as far as we can see in Nancy's peripheral blood, the evil cells have been wiped out. The only bad news about a four hundred WBC means that Nancy has little, if any, immunity left.

We have to be ever vigilant for infection, which is why Nancy can't have live flowers or fruits in her room. We also have to be very careful with visitors. And it's why I wash my hands so many times a day that they are as dry and as rough as sandpaper.

The rest of Nancy's blood count numbers are also good in comparison to her numbers upon admission. Her doctors were not exaggerating when they said she could easily have died in the first twenty-four hours. She was lucky to have received such prompt and competent attention.

Nancy also continues to receive a second chemotherapy drug, the pill ATRA, which I have nicknamed the "Parent" medicine.

Though a large part of Nancy's problem is too many of the white cells called myelocytes, the other part of the problem is that those white cells are immature and therefore don't function properly. ATRA helps new myelocytes grow up and mature. You may remember when Nancy started the ATRA, it caused fluid to form in her lungs, nearly requiring a transfer to the intensive care unit and, potentially, a respirator (which would have put me in the cardiac care unit, or CCU).

I am happy to report that since the first day's scare, Nancy is tolerating the ATRA. We look forward to hearing that like the Idarubicin, it is doing its job.

Summary: The chemotherapy is going well at this point, and Nancy has finished one of her meds for this first round.

One down, and many to go.

Best,

Winnie

The Power of a Letter

June 7, 11:02 p.m.

Dear Friends and Family,

So many of you have been sympathetic in your responses to my ramblings.

I am eternally grateful for your thoughts, prayers, and offers of help. In the middle of the night, when I watch Nancy sleeping, it is nice to have companions other than doubt and fear. Your notes and emails serve as confidantes in the dark of the late evening.

Thanks immensely.

Further, your stories about my bride give me new knowledge and bring smiles to my face.

An example:

Hi Nancy,

I don't know if you remember me, but we graduated from the University of Georgia together and started with TWA at the same time. We flew together from time to time and, as newbies, were always assigned to the back of the plane in E zone on full 747s!

I remember one trip to Madrid when you were working L5 and I was R5. A man in the last row gave you a really hard time and you came back to the galley crying. I knew it was nothing you did (you were the best flight attendant ever!), so I went back and told him off for making you cry. It turned out that his father had just died so he was upset and took it out on you. He ended up working the snack service in the galley for us while we delivered the sandwiches. Then he sent us each a pair of boots (he owned a shoe factory).

It's funny the stories you remember. In my many years of flying since, our Madrid trip was the only time any passenger ever sent me a present. But then, I can't remember ever working with a person like you before or since—fun, hardworking, and kind. I truly enjoyed those early days.

I hope your road to recovery is quick and painless. I don't know if you'd remember, but I met my husband of thirty-four years on my very first trip as a flight attendant en route to Shannon, Ireland. Unfortunately, he is going through chemo and radiation for lung cancer right now, so we understand your battle. I know you are surrounded by a loving family and wish you all the best.

Love,

Lee Waddell McCarthy

I was not surprised by my beloved's response when I read her that letter this morning. The rest of the day, she could only think and talk about what Lee was going through with her husband. She directed me to call Lee as soon as possible to offer my medical input.

Summary: Your many responses to Nancy's illness have been an incredible comfort during our tough moments and a true joy during our better days. I had not anticipated the breadth and depth of having Nancy's plight shared with so many. We have reconnected with a number of friends from the present and past, from near and far. All are now an integral part of Nancy's support team. Thanks for spreading the word.

Love,

Winnie

A Glimpse of Nancy's Garden

June 8, 3:03 a.m.

Dear Friends and Family,

Several of you have inquired about Nancy's mental health.

I've been asked time and again, "How is Nancy doing?" I assume the real and true meaning to the question is "How is Nancy dealing with a life-threatening illness? How is she feeling?"

I must admit, I've pondered this very issue many times.

Nancy is the most giving and selfless human being I have ever encountered. She is always thinking of others, not herself. And yet she is facing life's biggest mystery squarely in the eye.

How scared is she?

A little?

Somewhat?

Or just plain terrified?

Personally, I'm in the "terrified" category.

And is she depressed?

I am.

I ask myself over and over, "What more can I do? What can anyone do for that matter, and how can I facilitate it?"

Questions clatter in my head like the fast-moving balls of a pinball machine.

Nancy's father had a long, protracted battle with throat cancer that wasn't pretty. After his final surgery, he told Nancy, "I shouldn't have done it. It wasn't worth it."

Is Nancy having similar reflections about her treatment?

Will she talk to me about her private thoughts?

Her fears?

Her wishes?

I've always believed that Nancy and I were best friends and soul mates, able to tackle subjects tougher than the weather. But until last night, I've had quite honestly only fleeting glimpses of my wife's deepest feelings. While I'm single-handedly supporting the Kleenex industry, I've only seen Nancy cry once and that was about disrupting Jayna's Peru adventure.

Nancy has not wanted to discuss her disease, waving her hand and saying, "TMI (too much information)," when I wax medical. So I have surmised that she wants to process all that is happening to her silently and, for now, by herself.

I know this has to be a difficult time for her.

I hold her hand as much as she will allow.

Out of the blue, things changed this morning. For the first time, Nancy asked for her mobile phone.

"Hi, Mother, it's Nancy."

Leukemia has no effect on phonation. I suspect my mother-in-law knew her daughter's voice, even though it was their first conversation since Nancy's diagnosis.

"Yeah, they even have a nickname for me. I'm a 'leukie.'"

Humor. One of Nancy's primary MOs (and one that contributed to me falling head over heels for her). My tears contrasted her smile. Nancy's tone, her face, even the use of her free hand all gave the same message: *I am now able to talk about my disease. I am fine.*

"That's right, Mom. I guess you have to get 'the big C' to be admitted to the hospital these days. The 'big B' just isn't good enough to get above the ground floor."

Mary Lou, my mother-in-law, had recently taken an ambulance to the hospital for a bad back (the big B). She was sent home from the ER with a bunch of pills. Nancy's cancer (the big C), however, was the ticket for an extended hospital stay. Room 842 East, LDS Hospital, Salt Lake City—where Nancy finally called her other family members, talked with Jayna and Jaret about her disease, and told me she was ready for a "serious" discussion about the future.

I attribute Nancy's "opening up" to Jayna.

When Jayna arrived on the scene last week, one of her first comments was, "Daddy, didn't you notice that this room is dreary?" I wanted to tell her that I was too busy taking care of her mother to notice, but, truth be known, such details are not usually on my radar.

That is not the case with Jayna.

Last night, a new nurse was on duty. Nancy was napping when she entered the room and whispered, "Do you know what we nurses have nicknamed this room? 'The Garden.' We've never seen so many flowers. And look at the cards, balloons, and presents. Your wife must really be popular."

Our nurse was so right. The room display, plastic flowers and all, is but the tip of the iceberg. Calls, emails, letters, thoughts, and prayers continue to pour in like spring torrents in Utah. And it's been raining hard here, almost every day.

I remain astounded at the support and caring, and Nancy gets close to crying each time I read your correspondences to her. It is a great consolation to our entire family that so many of you are with us in spirit since Nancy is unable to have visitors and is too weak to talk much on the phone. Still there is no doubt your display of love is helping her endure the present and grapple with her future.

Summary: Nancy seems to be in a good place. I will update you again as my energy and emotions permit. Right now, both are in a good place, with the love of my life leading the charge.

Peace,

Winnie

A Kick to the Groin

June 11, 6:51 p.m.

Dear Friends and Family,

I've been working my daytime job during the hours that I'm not at the hospital these last few days, leaving me drained by the time Nancy's eyes close for an extended stretch, which in her world is two to three hours. I've been too exhausted to write.

Sorry.

Today, however, starts four much anticipated days off from the clinic.

In reality, there is a second reason I've waited to correspond.

Nancy's test results.

Yesterday, Nancy endured a procedure called a bone marrow biopsy. A large bore needle was inserted into the back of her pelvis to extract bone marrow tissue containing the parent cells that produce the various components of blood. Even though Dr. Morton used a local anesthetic, the technique is far from painless. The grinding sound of bone being crushed could be heard across the room. I cringed, even though I've done the procedure myself a few times during my medical training.

But you know my Nancy. Not a single sound or word was uttered when Dr. Morton thrust the needle deep into her bone. A barely felt squeeze of my hand and the slightest tensing of her eyebrows divulged that she was experiencing discomfort. In contrast, by the time I was wheeling her back to our room, I was drenched with sweat.

Once "home," Nancy immediately fell into a deep sleep; I presumed she was exhausted. Again, in comparison, I was wide-awake and fidgety. I walked the halls, pondering the coming hours. I faced a worry-filled, sleepless night. After all, the teaspoon of tissue-filled fluid Dr. Morton extracted from Nancy's back would soon tell us if the bone marrow killing medicine was doing its job. By tomorrow morning, Nancy's test results would be complete. We will know if Nancy has any prayer of beating her disease.

My bad night was nothing compared to Nancy's. Before the procedure, Nancy had taken several laps around the eighth-floor hallways, a proud smile hidden beneath her mask. She had laughed at my dumb jokes, eaten cookies topped with strawberry ice cream, and taken a long, hot shower. We enjoy simple things these days, and Nancy's shower culminated nearly forty-eight hours of her feeling pretty decent.

The good times ended for us three hours after the procedure; Nancy awoke from her slumber and sat straight up in her bed. Her face was flushed and she said her temples pounded and the ulcers in her mouth tingled. She struggled to find a less uncomfortable position. As I rang for the nurse, I put the back of my hand to Nancy's forehead. Our nurse confirmed my fear with her thermometer. Nancy was burning up with fever.

Nancy has had mild congestion since admission but is not allowed to blow her nose for fear of bleeding. As the night progressed, her congestion worsened, making breathing a chore. Between audible breaths, she pleaded, "Winnie, I ache." Inquiring where, she answered, "From the top of my head to the bottom of my feet." Nancy was miserable. Not only did my heart wrench with her pain, I was frantic.

Is this a bad omen for the test results?

I covered Nancy with blankets fresh from the warmer that sits at the end of our hallway. When the covers made her too hot, I took them off. I placed an ice bag on her neck and a second on her forehead. I wrapped her wrists in cold, wet wash-cloths and did the same to her elegant ankles. I rubbed her back softly, so as not to bruise. Nancy's oxygen level dropped below the safety zone and supplemental oxygen was restarted. I longed to see Nancy asleep, dreaming of better times. At least there was little time to fret over the bone marrow results.

This is the roller coaster of chemotherapy, and we have tried to relish the peaks. We know her condition can change quickly. And just like last time, it did.

By sunrise, the headache was gone, Nancy was weaned off of oxygen and back to room air, and her temperature was no more elevated than mine. By the time Dr. Russ Morton, our hematologist/oncologist, entered the room for his morning rounds, Nancy was sitting up in bed without squirming in pain.

Ready.

My heart rate increased as I noted the serious look on Russ's face and the way he wrinkled his brow. I took a very deep breath as he began to speak: "Nancy's bone marrow test revealed an empty marrow. This means we no longer see any cancer cells. The chemotherapy is working. It's as good as we could have hoped."

I silently cheered as his words penetrated my being. The "bad guy" cells had been wiped out by the "assassin" medicine. I nearly stood up and raised my fist like an Olympic athlete about to receive a gold medal. But Dr. Morton paused as he looked back at Nancy, and then me.

Why does he still look so serious?

Shouldn't we be planning a party?

Dr. Morton cleared his throat and continued: "However, we also received results from the tests we ran when Nancy was first admitted. The ones we ran to confirm our initial working diagnosis—the M3 type of leukemia. Unfortunately, they all came up the same. Nancy does *not* have the M3 type."

I sunk into my chair, wanting to vanish from the room. My head was spinning and my palms were so moist I had to rub them on my pants. I had been studying about leukemia during my sleepless nights. I knew what his next words would be before he spoke out loud.

"What this means is that Nancy's prognosis is not quite as good. We now think her classification is M5, but the exact type isn't important. We lump all non-M3 leukemias together. If you can achieve an initial remission like Nancy has, they have a cure rate between 30 to 40%."

His words felt like a kick to my groin. I wanted to throw up. Instead, I grabbed one of Nancy's elegant ankles and gently rubbed it. Nancy seemed to be handling it much better than me. Her facial expression hadn't changed. She was attentive and seemed to understand. She would later tell Jayna and me, "Don't worry, you two, everything will be all right. We'll adjust."

My expression did change; Dr. Morton had no trouble reading my feelings.

"I know this is disappointing, Winnie. And for good reason. This is a curve ball. A very tough curve ball. But despite this news . . . believe me . . . the sky is not falling."

Then why did it feel that way?

Dr. Morton went on to describe our next steps as I fought back my tears by biting my lip: Wait for Nancy's immunity to recover. About four more weeks, he thought. Then home for a two-week vacation. Then back in the hospital for another round of chemotherapy. Repeat the cycle several times. Each chemotherapy course would have the side effects we've come to expect: fevers, anemia, bruises, ulcers in the mouth, nausea, diarrhea, and generally feeling awful.

Each cycle would have a big risk—infection. Any bacteria, fungus, or virus smart enough to take advantage of her compromised state could mean game over.

Throughout, Nancy's face remained serene and beautiful. Flashing her amazingly warm smile, she thanked Dr. Morton as he departed through the door. She motioned me over for a kiss and followed it by stroking my hair.

How could she be comforting me?

I forced myself to rally and gave Nancy a long kiss too, not on her cheek as has become our recent habit, but on the lips.

Yes, our lives have once again been flipped upside down and sideways—but we are still spending the most intimate times a couple can spend together.

My new mantra will have to be "a 30–40% chance is better than 0%."

Isn't it?

Summary:

1. Nancy has achieved remission. For now, science can detect no trace of Nancy's AML. This is incredibly exciting, as good as we could have hoped. Your thoughts and prayers are working.

2. Nancy's road to a cure will be considerably longer and far tougher than we originally expected. Her diagnosis has changed from the more easily treated M3 subtype of AML to a non-M3 subtype of AML that often recurs with dire consequences. Still her current remission was achieved using only one induction (assassin) drug. Normally, two drugs are used in the beginning for a non-M3 AML. Though the change in diagnosis is truly depressing, we could have learned that besides not having the M3 subtype, Nancy also was not in remission. No remission would have meant disaster. Instead, she is in remission and will have multiple rounds of chemotherapy in an attempt to kill the leukemia cells that remain hidden and undetectable by current testing methods.

My very best,

Winnie

A New Perspective
June 11, 11:08 p.m.

Dear Friends and Family,

Well, as you might surmise from the previous letter, I have been feeling sorry for myself today. Just when I thought I couldn't possibly bear to see pain etched across Nancy's face again—or just when I wondered how I would make Jaret feel safe, or just when I wondered how I could convince Jayna to be twenty-two years old again (her first reaction to the new information was "I guess I won't be going back to college")—I discovered our newest neighbors on the eighth (cancer) floor: a family who has given me *the gift of perspective*.

As part of my daily routine, I had ventured to the cafeteria to get Nancy two large scoops of strawberry ice cream and was heading back to the eighth floor. I often take the stairs, but for some reason, I took the elevator back "home" because I needed to get there quickly. My excuse? I didn't want the ice cream to melt. In reality, I was simply too weary for the nine flights of stairs from the basement restaurant. (These are the "rationalization" games I sometimes play to get through the day.)

When the elevator stopped on the ground floor, a man and woman in their midforties walked into the elevator. In an instant, I realized that they looked familiar. I actually knew them—Kevin and Marie. I had been their family's doctor on and off for years and Marie was a friend of Nancy's. In fact, Jayna had been in a play with one of the family's two daughters. It was an awkward moment as we exchanged greetings.

Should I ask why they are here?
Should I tell them why I am here?

Before I could decide, Marie said, "Winnie, I've heard about Nancy's illness. I am so sorry."

My normal reaction, tears welling up and a momentary inability to speak, kicked in. I looked at the floor. Finally, lifting my head up I recovered enough composure to respond, "Thanks, Marie. What brings you and your family here?" (Fortunately, I didn't say, "This late and after normal visiting hours.")

I was stunned by Marie's answer: "You probably remember our oldest daughter Megan. You took care of her when she was growing up. She just graduated from college in Virginia and came home for the summer. Megan has just been transferred from the recovery room after ten hours of surgery. She is on the same floor as Nancy."

I thought to myself, *"Why is she on the cancer floor?"*

After a brief momentary pause, Marie continued and I learned the answer: "Megan started having stomach pains two weeks ago. It turns out she has ovarian cancer."

My legs nearly buckled under me, but fortuitously we arrived at the eighth floor and the ding of the elevator gave us all a needed break as we exited. Marie continued after the elevator door closed: "It's pretty bad, Winnie. They had to remove her right ovary, part of her bowel, part of her bladder, and part of her liver. The cancer had spread everywhere." Marie's tears matched those of Kevin. I gave them both a hug, trying to hide my own wet face.

As I walked to Nancy's room, I realized how selfish I have been with our family's plight. Megan is a mere twenty-two years old. She faces drugs with horrible side effects at best and more painful surgeries at worst. She has a prognosis far more grave than Nancy's, probably less than a 1% chance of reaching the age of twenty-five. My heart broke into little pieces and I wanted to curse a supreme being, if he or she exists. How could this happen to someone so young and so full of promise? It took over ten minutes to regain my composure before delivering Nancy's ice cream.

"You must have walked up those steps, Winnie," Nancy chided. "It's almost melted."

I didn't explain—at least for now.

Instead, I hugged Nancy more tightly than usual, hoping not to cause bruises.

Nancy's spirit is strong and mine is regaining its vigor. During the good hours, we laugh and kid each other, and I tell her of the incredible energy coming from your direction. She is upbeat and positive.

I will write more soon, next time, with any luck, from a view at the top of a summit on our continuing roller coaster ride. I hope this letter hasn't been too negative. Tonight, I gained new perspective and thought it might help to share it with you.

There is a bright side to this experience: Our daughter has arrived safely home. Our son is doing well. I am able to feel the strength of family relationships as never before. And with regard to our friends, I am truly astounded at how lucky we are each and every day.

I had no idea so many people care about and love Nancy.

Summary: Despite our setback, Nancy sees more light than darkness. I have a new perspective, and am trying to see things through the lens of Nancy's eyes.

All my love,

Winnie

A Half-Full Glass of Lemonade

June 18, 3:36 p.m.

Dear Friends and Family,

My mother was an optimistic, completely positive person. I grew up amid phrases like "Make lemons into lemonade" and "The glass is always half full." Though she died several years ago, her long ago guidance has been vital for these challenging times.

A week ago, my sister-in-law Linda called from Georgia. I nearly dropped the phone when she announced, "Winnie, from the minute Nancy entered the hospital, I've been working to free up my schedule. I really want to see Nancy and help you, Jaret, and Jayna. I bought my ticket today. Can you pick me up at the airport tomorrow afternoon?"

Speechless, I paused to gather my thoughts. How could I tell her "NO" gently? I replied, "Jayna and I are doing great, considering everything. We alternate times at the hospital. Jaret has adjusted to Nancy being in the hospital. My partners, along with everyone else at work, have been totally supportive. There has been an unbelievable outpouring from friends locally—even as far away as New Zealand. Everyone wants to help. So for right now, Linda, we're actually all right."

I really wanted to say, "Don't come now. We don't need you." Or more accurately, "We're not ready yet."

Linda ignored my request and informed me, "Anyway, I land at 2:40 in the afternoon, Winnie. After you check your schedule, let me know if I should call a cab."

As is too often the case, I was all too wrong.

Linda arrived and has been a whirlwind of activity ever since. She fills in at the hospital when I am working and Jayna has a commitment such as her appointment at the University of Utah. She picks up garbage bags for the compactor. She has restocked our home refrigerator with real food. She does things like noticing that our houseplants are drooping like they're living in a desert. And most importantly, she is taking Jaret under her wing.

I see evidence of her presence everywhere I look in Woodland. Actually, the first several days she was here, I rarely saw Linda because she has slept at the hospital with Jayna on the "every other night" schedule when I didn't sleep in Nancy's room. Nancy glowingly described it to me this morning as a "girls' night in." Even during the days when I am in Salt Lake City with Nancy, Linda has been busy being "Aunt-in-Chief."

So when I don't see Jaret in nearly three days, I ask Linda the same question many of you sympathetically ask me: "How's Jaret doing?" I spend the day at work and go directly to the hospital to relieve Jayna for my "sleepover" with Nancy.

"Jaret's fine. He and I . . ." and then she tells me of the many adventures she and Jaret have had the day before at the market, the toy store, or the park. She talks about his coursework, which she is now monitoring.

"In fact, Jaret and I have been talking and he has something to tell you. I thought I'd bring him here this afternoon after his classes. He wants to see you and his mom."

When I returned from lunch in the hospital cafeteria today, Nancy was nearly asleep and Jaret was sitting on the rollaway bed engrossed in his Gameboy. He looked totally connected to Linda, whose shoulder was serving as a pillow for his head. Linda nodded at me and gently nudged him, "J, your dad is here."

As sometimes occurs when Jaret is excited, he skipped the perfunctory "Hellos" and "How are yous" and burst into conversation about what was on his mind.

"You know, Dad. Mom has always done everything for me since I was a baby."

Jaret's assessment is accurate. Nancy has helped him with everything from daily living activities to his studies. She has been his chauffeur since Jaret doesn't have a driver's license. Most importantly, she has been his emotional bedrock. She has continuously showered him with the unconditional love necessary to build his self-esteem. But today, he showed the fruits of her years as a Super Mom.

"It's my turn, Dad. I need to learn how to take care of Mom. Tell me what to do."

This evening I treated Linda and Jayna to a special dinner. Jaret didn't join us as he decided to stay with his mother. It was our first meal in a long time not consumed at the hospital cafeteria. I couldn't help but notice the look of satisfaction plainly revealed across Jaret's face. It was the same look he exhibited when he announced his intention to assume a more active role with his mom.

As we walked out the door, I heard Jaret ask, "Can I get you some cold water, Mom?"

Summary: My sister-in-law Linda has arrived in Utah to assist our family. She made me very aware that our glass is more than half full and, in fact, contains lemonade.

Much love,

Winnie

As Close to Heaven as You Can Get

June 19, 11:50 p.m.

Dear Friends and Family,

When the elevator door opened this afternoon, I was shocked to see so many people. A thirtysomething male carrying his lunch tray from the basement cafeteria studied my face: "Don't be shy. We'll make room."

I secured a spot in the left front corner of the "car" while I analyzed the scene and realized the answer. Surprisingly, this was the first time I had arrived at the hospital during lunch, the middle of posted "visiting hours." In contrast, I usually arrive early in the morning or deep into the night. During the majority of my rides I am alone, able to make funny faces with impunity to the mirrors composing the elevator walls.

The packed elevator stopped at every single floor. Anxious fathers departed to the obstetrics floor. An athletic-appearing woman exited to the orthopedic wing. Middle-aged sons and daughters rushed to the internal medicine floor.

By the time the door closed on the seventh floor, a fortyish female was my only companion. Her tall, thin frame was slightly hunched, as if she was carrying the weight of the world. I couldn't help but notice bloodshot, puffy eyes. Her facial expression resembled what I assume someone would look like while being stuck with needles underneath each of her fingernails—pained.

Noticing my gaze, she looked downward. Similar to her eyes, mine were also red and swollen. As is typical, the trip down the mountain from Park City to the hospital had included my daily cry. The woman nodded. I was an accepted member of the fraternity.

"You going to the eighth, too?" she asked softly. "Never thought I'd dread visiting a penthouse."

Floor number eight, the penthouse of this hospital, is the "cancer floor."

Nearest to heaven?

The woman and I disembarked in silence. And I did not make a funny face in the mirror today.

Since it was midday, I stopped in Room 801, now "home" to Megan, the twenty-two-year-old Park City girl with advanced ovarian cancer, whom I wrote about a few days ago. I hesitated a few moments and then carefully wiped my eyes before entering her room.

Summary: As I wax poetic, I sometimes find metaphors in my new daily life. I am plagued by unanswerable questions. The final stop on the elevator is the penthouse (eighth) floor where Nancy and my young friend, Megan, reside. It is closest to heaven.

So much love,

Winnie

Cherishing Each Day as It Comes

June 20, 11:07 p.m.

Dear Friends and Family,

Today was a *great* day.

Nancy feels good. She no longer has a fever, and is, for her, full of energy after receiving transfusions of red blood cells and platelets. For the first time in days, we ventured down the eighth-floor hall and were "outside" our room for nearly an hour before lunch. She devoured everything on her tray and within minutes, was snoring again in a sound, nonrestless slumber. For the entire day, Room 842 was filled with Nancy's brilliance. My face aches from constant smiling.

Oh, and I've saved the best reason for last.

Midafternoon, Dr. Prystas, one of our cancer doctors, made an unexpected visit, sporting a smile as big as a half-moon. "Nancy, we're seeing the early signs of bone marrow recovery in your blood tests. It won't be long before you're able to go home for a few weeks before the next round."

A "vacation" in Woodland on the not-too-distant horizon? OMG!

So Nancy and I are doing great. Which means it is probably a good time to catch up on everyone else.

In addition to the frequent questions of "How is Jaret doing?" and "Anything I can do to help Jaret?" A few of you have asked, "Is Jaret aware of the seriousness of Nancy's illness?"

(Thank you, by the way, for always asking about Jaret.)

The answer is YES. He has even formed his own unique insight.

After the change in diagnosis nine days ago when I was melancholic, Jaret walked over to my chair and gave me a hug. As usual, his declaration was short and to the point: "I'm still optimistic, Dad. I know Mom could kick the bucket, but I have a good feeling." Jaret had regrouped for the continued battle well before I had in a moment of self-indulgent self-absorption.

And what about Jayna?

Jayna has just redecorated our hospital "home" for the third time. Also, she and her mom have begun religiously watching reruns of a TV series that gives me pause: *Six Feet Under.* And it's all I need to hear for me to go to the cafeteria or take a quick bike ride.

So at this point, I believe, the kids are fine. They are certainly a huge comfort, not only to Nancy but to me as well.

The final question I want to address tonight also originates from a large number of you.

"Nancy's in remission?" is a question I've heard countless times. The emphasis is always on the word "remission" and the higher pitch assigned to that last word seems to me to convey an element of doubt. I suspect Nancy's plight has led to the confusion.

For most of us, remission paints a pretty picture: Nancy feeling great, going home, being "normal"—even if it is recognized that a remission may not last forever.

Allow me to clarify.

CR, or complete remission in the world of leukemia, means the cancer cells have disappeared. Indeed, as many of you know, last week Nancy once again had a large bore needle jammed into her hipbone to perform the bone marrow test, the one that looks at the blood-forming tissues of the body. The results were exciting beyond belief. After only a few chemotherapy treatments and in less than two weeks, her bone marrow was "empty." No leukemic cells were detected—CR. The doctors, nurses, lab technicians, respiratory technicians, as well as the clerks, janitors, and other hospital personnel who know Nancy, all congratulated us on achieving remission. They recognize *big* news. If she hadn't achieved CR, the future would be darker than nighttime in a cavern without chambers.

However, chemotherapy is indiscriminate. It is not unusual to call the "chemo" drugs poisons. Though I nicknamed them "assassin" medicines, "poisons" may be more accurate.

When chemotherapy works like it has for Nancy, it is supposed to kill all the leukemic cells in her bone marrow. However, the few normal white cells left perish with the "bad guy" leukemic white cells. The parent cells that create new red blood cells, the cells that transport oxygen through our bloodstream, are also destroyed. The platelets, the particles in charge of bleeding prevention, are additionally demolished by the indiscriminate power of the chemotherapy drugs.

Consequently, even though Nancy is technically in remission, she is nearly as sick as the day she arrived—about three weeks ago today. She is anemic. She is at risk for serious bleeding into one of her vital organs. And even scarier, she has severely impaired immunity and therefore is susceptible to both common and unusual infections.

With her bone marrow wiped out, Nancy feels totally debilitated and extremely weak. She remains in isolation in a special room designated only for immunocompromised patients, awaiting her body's normal blood-forming capacity to bounce back. She remains alive courtesy of red blood cell transfusions to help her anemia and platelet transfusions to prevent bleeding. What's more, Nancy is taking a wide variety of antibiotics and antiviral drugs to prevent infection, the biggest worry.

Yes, Nancy is in remission. But she is still *very* sick.

I hope my explanation makes sense. If not, please ask me specific questions. I'll try again.

And please know that there are good hours, afternoons, and, even days (like today) when Nancy is posttransfusions and feels better.

We cherish each day as it comes to us.

Summary: Great news! Nancy has achieved CR, or complete remission.

With love,

Winnie

Only in the South

June 21, 12:02 a.m.

Dear Friends and Family,

In the last update, I described Nancy's lab results and how they made her feel physically. However, I realize I didn't answer the most frequent and important question that continues to be asked now that we've been in the hospital over three weeks: "How are Nancy's emotions holding up?"

Some emotions seem obvious, even though Nancy has not yet expressed them. Nancy has to be sad. Who wouldn't be? And if I had to bet, she is scared. Is she angry? Or more than sad, depressed? I see occasional glimpses of these emotions, but I oftentimes wonder if I am projecting my own feelings.

Each day I leave the door open to connect on a deeper level. I ask, "What's on your mind today, my love?" I inquire time and again, "What can I do?" Many of you have expressed helplessness in relation to Nancy's situation. Powerlessness and vulnerability are emotions that have a constant presence in my emotional wheelhouse.

I hold Nancy's hand. I tell my newest silly story in a feeble attempt to provoke laughter. And I catalogue into a daily summary all the thoughts and prayers that you are sending in her direction. But even between the closest of individuals, infinite distance exists. I can only hope to occasionally bridge the gap.

My best guess? Nancy is doing as well as can be expected. Having cancer is a horrible plight. Sitting next to it isn't great either.

Perhaps a few stories will give the best answer (and insight) to your question.

On her morning rounds, Dr. Prystas (one of our cancer doctors), told Nancy, "You need to eat more if you can. Nutrition is important to our fight. I'll write an order. They should give you whatever you want to eat whenever you want it."

Dr. Prystas had barely shut the door when Nancy announced, "If you see the dietician, tackle her."

The same plea went to the nurse, the intern, and our now familiar cleaning lady. Nancy is ready for the foods she likes, anything to combat the nausea and general lousiness of chemotherapy. It was also a full-hearted statement to all of us around her. Nancy seems eager to participate in her care. She is like a teenaged girl readying for a date, and her desire to get better is growing stronger.

In context, Nancy's "tackle her" statement is even more amazing. Nancy is from the Deep South. Georgia, to be specific. As a "Yankee," it took me years to understand how southerners communicate.

Southerners are rarely direct. My mother-in-law can spend a whole afternoon discussing dinner instead of just saying, "Let's eat."

Nancy is not as extreme. However, when she asks, "Do you think I should wear my navy coat," I'm off the hook. She will be decked in navy; I just need to agree.

"Are you tired?" is southern for "I'm tired now. Can we go to bed?"

So instead of saying, "If you see the dietician, let me know," Nancy's "tackle the dietician" is completely out of character. Her response illustrates a strong will.

Thank goodness.

A second story.

"It hit me hard today, Winnie. I can't believe I'll have to do this chemotherapy thing again. Three more times. I feel like crap."

What could I possibly say? It had been a bad day for Nancy. The phlebotomist who normally draws Nancy's blood was off, and her replacement "missed" the first two times. She had to stand to have a chest X-ray even though she felt particularly weak. And she had to give three different urine specimens. By late morning, fever and chills were return visitors to Room 842. Nancy had no energy to walk. She even turned down her daily shower, too tired to make another trip to her bathroom.

"You know, Nancy, the day before yesterday, when Chuck and I took our mountain bike ride, we went on a brand new trail in Round Valley. It was really hard for me. But yesterday, we rode the same trail. And it wasn't so bad. Actually, it was almost easy. Your treatments will be like that."

Nancy grabbed my hand between both of hers. There were fewer wrinkles on her forehead than moments before. Her eyes spoke volumes and I couldn't speak. I didn't need to. For once, I chose the correct words. She smiled, closed her eyes, and fell asleep.

Your emails and cards have the same soothing effect.

I once again send our thanks.

For both of us.

A final story.

Jayna ordered five hats from the American Cancer Society catalog. They were delivered yesterday. When I arrived today, Nancy was wearing the pink one. She wore matching lipstick and was also sporting earrings given to Nancy by our dear friend Mona for their magic healing power. I even detected eyeliner, mascara, and a hint of blush. Today Nancy looked more beautiful than ever.

Many years ago, one of my medical school mentors taught me the importance of "accepting one's disease." When I gave Nancy a longer-than-usual kiss and told her how ravishing she was, she removed the hat. Her recently shaved, glistening bald head only added to the magnificence.

After saying "Wow" and showering her head with kisses and soft caresses, I asked, "Why now?"

Her twinkling eyes complimented the mischievous tone of her voice when she replied, "It was time."

I suspect Nancy was talking about more than her clean-shaven head.

I expect as Nancy gains strength that you will hear from her.

Summary: As best I can tell; Nancy is doing as well emotionally as can be expected.

> With much love from my
> bald and beautiful wife
> (and me),
>
> Winnie

Playing the Waiting Game

June 23, 11:29 a.m.

Dear Friends and Family,

Three days ago, I wrote that our medical team thought that Nancy's immune system was on the rebound.

They were wrong.

Nancy's immune status remains unchanged, and the last two days have been less than great because the anticipated rise in the level of her white blood cells has not yet occurred. White blood cells are the cells that fight infections.

Nancy's fevers have become more frequent and her temperature levels are higher. Our medical team has concluded that an unwanted enemy has more than likely gained a foothold. An infectious disease consultant has been recruited to help find the exact spot and type of germ, as well as to manage the many different anti-infectious agents Nancy is now receiving.

I wish I could report better news. My heart is full of agony.

A few hours ago, I was sitting on the bed, holding Nancy's delicate hand. Most of her bruises have faded, deep purple replaced by faint blue. Nancy made a soft, guttural sound indicating she was pleased that I was gently stroking each finger. Her skin was not so hot as it was an hour earlier and her face was calm, the hint of a smile on her lips. I thought she might be dreaming. I even found myself wondering if her spirit could be in a better place, far away from tubes and needles, bells and buzzers, pills and tests.

Unexpectedly, Nancy's entire body twitched and I nearly fell off the bed's edge as I jumped backward by reflex. She opened her eyes and I was mesmerized by the blue sparkle, as bright as the day we met more than two and a half decades ago. Once Nancy closed her eyes again, my mind drifted back to that fateful August day during the summer of 1978 when Nancy walked into the medical clinic at Mammoth Hot Springs in Yellowstone National Park.

Though it was a sun-filled day outside, "lightning" struck me in that exam room so many years ago. Nancy's soft voice and ready smile instantly made me feel like we were old friends. I almost forgot everything as we exchanged initial pleasantries. From that very first second, I was drawn into Nancy's gaze. Her eyes were the color of the summer sky on a cloudless day. They exuded the warmth of that season. Nancy's smile was full, kind, and part of an expression that was both deep and inviting. I remember reacting to my feelings with nervousness, and I'm sure I acted like an intern interviewing his first patient. My heart raced, my hands were clammy, and I stuttered more than once as if my mouth wasn't connected to my brain.

Once the visit was complete, I walked Nancy into the waiting room, trying to figure out what I could do to prevent her from driving off in the late afternoon sunset and out of my life.

"What are you doing tonight?" I sheepishly inquired. "Would you be interested in experiencing an authentic cowboy town? Gardiner, Montana, is just a bit north of us." Such brashness was completely out of character in my normal interactions and, looking back, even further "on the edge" given that I had met Nancy as a patient.

It turned out Nancy was struck by the same "lightning" bolt.

To my surprise and delight, she answered, "I'd love to . . ."

Subsequently, we spent a magical night talking about life, love, politics, religion, and most of all, each other. Our first date ended as the sun rose, and we continued our friendship and subsequent romance for many months by phone. (Mobile phones didn't exist back then, so we had triple-digit long distance bills.)

Six months later, having physically spent only twelve days together (because she was living in Boston and I was residing in Yellowstone and then Park City), we tied the knot. Our friends and family thought we were crazy. They were right. As they say, "All the rest is history." And that was over twenty-seven years ago.

Just as I finished my soliloquy, Nancy opened her eyes again. "Did I fall asleep?" she asked me.

It's the time of day when Nancy is weak. Her tiredness can mean her blood count is so low that she needs another transfusion. Or that the wrong combination of her ever-increasing list of medicines is making her loopy. Or that her temperature is elevated. Sometimes it means that her oxygen needs adjusting. Each condition alone can sap her dwindling reserves and make it a Herculean effort for her to just open her eyes. In Nancy's case, several of these conditions often are in play at the same moment.

About an hour ago, Nancy experienced a "rigor," the violent shaking that occurs when the body attempts to lose heat during a rapid temperature spike. Some of us have seen our children do it. Nancy is not a child. Our kind and competent nurse, Becky, was visibly flustered when she pulled the thermometer from Nancy's ear.

"Forty degrees Celsius! Oh! I'll call the doctor."

"Isn't that 104 Fahrenheit?" I cried.

It didn't matter. Nancy's temperature was high—extremely high and a reflection of the silent battle somewhere in her increasingly fragile body. Becky left the room and I was left holding Nancy tight, tears streaming down my face.

"It's all right, Winnie." Nancy told me between chattering teeth.

I felt powerless. Inept.

I'm a doctor, aren't I?

I held Nancy ever tighter while Becky returned with Tylenol and more ice. Ten minutes passed, and Nancy fell once again into an exhausted sleep.

Nancy didn't move for the next hour or so as I sat and watched her chest rise and fall. I visualized for her. I imagined waves sneaking up a white sand beach touching Nancy's toes as she lay on a towel, basking in the bright sunshine. The air smelled salty and fresh from the breeze off the ocean. It was a pleasant contrast to our sterile hospital room. I hoped my thoughts were transmitted into Nancy's dream. It was so peaceful on the beach.

Nancy's eyes opened again, "You didn't answer me. Did I fall asleep?"

I nodded and stroked her forehead.

"I'm sorry, Winnie. I can't believe I did that. I'm just so tired."

"Don't be sorry, love. It's much better when you fall asleep in the middle of your sentence than in the middle of mine."

We both laughed and I kissed the soft stubble above her forehead.

Nancy's immunity is severely suppressed. The chemotherapy that killed the leukemia, or "bad guy," cells has also killed the ones she needs to fight off normal and unusual infections. Her situation is akin to "friendly fire." Without one type of white blood cells called neutrophils, it is common for a germ to attack. Our medical team is now in full mobilization to find the infection and adjust her drugs appropriately.

Just now, Nancy has endured a procedure called a "bronchoscopy." A tube was inserted down her throat and into her lungs and samples were taken.

In between fevers, Nancy and I are now able to talk and even laugh. But the easiest way for me to see a smile on her face is to read her the news all of you share with us.

We wait and we hope.

Summary: Nancy is much sicker than the last time I wrote. Fortunately, she is lucid and not in pain. Though her vital signs remain stable, she is requiring more oxygen.

Thanks all for your hopes
and prayers,

Winnie

Beauty Is in the Eye of the Beholder

June 23, 10:10 p.m.

Dear Friends and Family,

After this morning's update, I thought it best to lighten the mood with a story I've been meaning to relate to you.

"I'm going to be bald and beautiful," Nancy declared out of the blue.

Though there is no doubt about the latter, the former has not seemed to be part of the picture. Then, all of a sudden last week, Nancy's hair started falling out in clumps. For the longest time, we have been waiting, even expecting, this side effect from chemotherapy. Still, until Nancy's statement, we have disregarded the inevitable.

In lots of ways, I am reminded of fall in the Utah Mountains, when I know snow is imminent. "Maybe this year it won't snow until February," I tell myself. "It was nearly seventy degrees today." I know my logic is clouded by my desire for one last mountain bike ride on trails covered with fallen yellow aspen leaves, making them look like the Yellow Brick Road in *The Wonderful Wizard of Oz*. Then, the next morning, I awaken to two feet of white stuff and I'm searching the back of my closet looking for my warmest coat.

Many of you know that Nancy is a behind-the-scenes, seemingly laid-back kind of woman. She is always the one to stay and clean up after events. She organizes those around her, like me, in her all-encompassing southern style. "Maybe we should do the dishes real fast before we leave," she whispers in my ear. (Translation: Start helping with the dishes if you want to get home tonight.)

It should not be surprising, then, to hear what happened to Nancy's stylish blondish locks. I was at work and called Jayna, who had just returned from a run to the cafeteria.

"How's Mom doing?" I asked, first thing first as always.

Jayna is a saint like her mom. She pretends not to mind me calling every hour or so on the days I am at work.

"Different."

I clutched the phone tightly, fearing the worst.

"What do you mean, Jayna?"

Jayna's mischievous giggle tickled my ear and soothed my anxiety.

"I can't believe it, Dadder. She did it while I was gone. Rebecca (one of our favorite certified nursing assistants) shaved Mom's head. But she doesn't look like Charles Barkley, like she hoped. She looks even better."

And so it was that Nancy jumped into the fray, proudly proclaiming her arrival into the fraternity (or sorority, for that matter) of chemotherapy patients. Was her head shiny? A bump or lump here or there? Resolving bruises? I could hardly wait to see.

So why am I giving you details of an event I mentioned in a previous update?

I simply want to finish the details I omitted about Jaret.

As I alluded to you in previous notes, when Jaret was younger, he'd close his eyes as we passed a cemetery on the way to school. Part of his condition is a near phobia about bones and blood and most things medical. Why he chose me for a dad, I don't know, but his mother has protected him well over the years from anything predictably unpleasant—like the bald head of a cancer patient.

Hence you can imagine the shock when Jaret entered the room and found his mom—hairless. Not surprisingly, Nancy was not wearing one of her many new hats (deepest thanks for those who have expanded her wardrobe) because of her fevers and resultant need to lose body heat.

"Uh, Mom . . . Uh, uh, what happened?"

"Oh, Jaret, I am so sorry. I forgot to tell you. I meant to wear a hat when you visited."

Jaret didn't scream. He didn't run out the door. He didn't do anything but hold his mom's hand, and then he carefully touched the stubble that used to be long and soft and pretty.

"Uh, it looks good, Mom. You're still beautiful."

Though Jaret didn't cry in the room, when I drove him back to his dorm room at Westminster College, he did shed a few tears. "Do you think Mom misses her hair?"

For some questions, I have no answers.

Summary: I knew I could find at least one positive amid today's sobering events. Jaret is growing up daily.

Love from Jaret, Jayna,
the bald lady and me,

Winnie

It's All or Nothing

June 24, 11:06 p.m.

Dear Friends and Family,

"What's my prognosis, Winnie?"

The question didn't emanate from Nancy, though Nancy and I occasionally discuss such things now. Instead speaking was Megan, the twenty-two-year-old ovarian cancer patient from Park City who is residing just down the hall from Nancy.

Today's visit was different.

It was just Megan and me in the room. The postsurgical NG (nasogastric) tube has been removed from Megan's nose and she was celebrating by sending her parents out to dinner so that she could watch *Law and Order* in solitude.

I'd attempted to leave, but Megan asked that I sit next to her "for a bit." After I explained Nancy's disease, including the disappointing change in diagnosis that lowered her odds to 30–40% from the original 70%, Megan looked me straight in the eye and posed that tough question. There was no place for me to hide.

Momentarily, I was speechless.

What could I say to this vibrant young woman, a college graduate of only three weeks?

What words could I craft for someone whose bright future and full life has been redressed in the darkest of colors?

What had her doctors told her?

Her parents?

"Megan, I don't know the details of your disease. And, to be honest, I don't want to know"—like with my Nancy, I sometimes choose not to ask questions or to search the medical literature—"With cancer, sometimes you don't want to think too far in the future. For example, if Nancy needs a bone marrow transplant, her sister and brother are the logical donors. But I don't want to know yet if one of them is a match. I will only want to know when we are forced in that direction. So I have to tell you that I don't know the specifics of your prognosis . . . on purpose."

My too-young friend nodded her head, acknowledging understanding, and I found myself marveling at her long, thick, ink-black hair. Her locks flowed onto her shoulders at the top of her hospital gown like the splash of a waterfall, the ends seeming to curl upward like water hitting a rock. I wondered if she was aware that she would soon be joining Nancy's fraternity (or is it a sorority?). I wondered how she would feel about being bald. At least I would have the opportunity to tell her she was beautiful.

"That said, your prognosis . . . your numbers . . . they only matter on paper. You are young. You are strong. You are a fighter. Whether your doctors tell you that you have a 90% chance or a 9% chance, for you as one individual—it is all or nothing. Your chance is either 0% or 100%. Many people love Nancy, so I've received countless emails and letters. Several have included stories about patients given little or no chance who did beat the odds. For example, one of Nancy's oldest friends, Annie Alfano from Connecticut, has a son; his name is Eric. He was born with Down's syndrome and at six developed leukemia like Nancy. The doctors told his mother that he only had an 18% chance of surviving. I'm happy to tell you that Eric just celebrated his seventeenth birthday. Megan, the next few months will not be easy. But you are surrounded by love and will have lots of help. You can do it."

Megan gave me the largest of smiles as a single tear ran down her left cheek. She sunk back into the many pillows on her bed, her entire body seeming to relax. I kissed her forehead and walked out the door. The tear on my left cheek matched hers.

Now that's perspective.

My little angel, Megan, all 102 pounds of her, will be discharged from the hospital tomorrow. When her surgical scars are healed in the next few weeks, she will begin aggressive chemotherapy. Her father tells me the latest news is favorable. Most of her cancer was removed by the surgery, so they are hoping the medicine will kill the remaining tumor. Please save a thought or prayer for her.

Summary: Our fellow Park City neighbor is doing better and will go home tomorrow. We are hoping that she will inhabit the small percentage of her disease's survival rate that does well.

With more love than
I knew I possessed,

Winnie

The Answer Is "Super"

June 26, 2:50 a.m.

Dear Friends and Family,

Besides worrying about Nancy, besides inquiring about Jaret and Jayna, many of you have posed the same question to me the past twenty-eight days.

The question "How are *you*?" has made its way into many of your emails, notes, and letters.

In all honesty, I have been less than direct in my answers. With Nancy lying so sick, how can I describe my sadness, my terror, and my anger?

My guts have churned in turmoil.

My thoughts have railed against demons.

My emotions change as rapidly as Nancy's temperature.

How can I possibly describe the way I feel?

As a doctor, I often know too much. As the spouse of a soul mate with a complicated life-threatening disease, I know too little. Too many times, the closest one-word description is "horror." But even that term sometimes seems extremely inadequate.

My basket full of feelings doesn't easily translate into words, so I've hidden them from you as much as possible in order to provide care for Nancy—and support for Jaret and Jayna. In reality, I don't know that I've done a good job of either the hiding or the caring.

In an unexpected way, it has been very hard to realize that you care so deeply about Nancy and me. I struggle with the concept of Nancy and myself—on display. Should I tell you everything? Nancy and I talk at almost any hour on the nights

91

we spend together in Room 842. Whenever she wakens or is awakened by the staff, I make myself accessible.

Our conversations are often short now because Nancy tires easily, but our topics are not those of daily conversation. By this point in our journey, they are intimate. Nancy has affirmed that she is generally satisfied with her life. I always hoped that was the case, but now all doubts have disappeared. Three nights ago, she sat up straight in her bed and out of nowhere declared to me that she is definitely "at peace" and has very few regrets. Of course, a big part of why she told me was so she could ask if I felt the same way. She followed her revelation with, "I am worried about you, Winnie."

Nancy may wish that she had not made her sister eat dirt when they were kids or that she had handled an issue or two differently with Jaret or Jayna—but those types of things are pretty trivial in the big picture of nearly fifty-seven years on this planet. Last night at around 2 a.m. she went a step further: "Winnie, it's important to me that you know how I feel. I've been extremely lucky in my life. I'm comfortable with whatever the future holds." Direct, non-southern speak. We held each other for a long, long time.

Nancy has expressed to me that she hates to see others, especially ones we care so much about, "fussing" on our behalf. Don't take this wrongly. The thought of losing my soul mate is the toughest challenge I have ever faced; still, I know that Nancy, I, and each of you will leave this earth in due time. Even as I write, I have two other friends facing equally life-threatening battles.

Sometimes it simply feels weird and uncalled for that you, our dearest of friends, have offered so many kind words, thoughts, and deeds. Nancy and I can't help but feel surrounded by your love; except there are times we feel overwhelmed and even unworthy. And I continue to think of Megan, my angel friend, with ovarian cancer at twenty-two. Her plight is truly a tragedy and one difficult to rationally understand. Ours is personally sad and devastating, but Nancy has lived a full and fruitful life. In our situation, Nancy and I may merely be facing the inevitable ebb and flow of life's forces.

Please don't think for one millisecond that I don't want to battle this leukemia to win a few more days, weeks, months, or even years with my beloved Nancy. Or that I wouldn't trade places so she could continue to be "Super Mom" to Jaret and Jayna, the special light to her friends, or the incredible human being she is to the many others she has touched during her life. I will support Nancy and persuade her to fight as hard as she can for as many months or years as necessary.

As long as she is not suffering.

As long as there is reasonable hope.

I share these somewhat random thoughts so you can understand my reticence in addressing directly your simple question, "How are you?"

It is no wonder then that these three simple words, "How are you?" keep me awake many nights. I have always been a positive person. Why not? I live in a wonderful place, have a satisfying job, and, yes, I have a magnificent wife and children.

So for as long as I can remember, my customary reply to "How are you?" has usually been *"Super."*

Short.

Positive.

Efficient.

And though probably not listened to by the questioner, my answer has been an accurate reflection of how I most often feel—at least until twenty-eight days ago, when my world dramatically changed.

In guilt and sometimes between tears, I end up revealing my sadness. Perfect strangers sometimes end up crying with me. I constantly struggle about whom and how much information I can or should share. I still haven't mastered these questions and perhaps never will.

We're only amid the first skirmish in a long fight against leukemia. But one thing has become clear. I often feel selfish when so many others have problems equally pressing. I'm supposed to be the helper, right? But at least for this one day, at least for the next twelve hours before some new lab test or negative development occurs, I am ready to scream the answer.

To friends.

To acquaintances.

To people I don't even know.

I have finally returned to my one-word, familiar reply to the omnipresent question of "How are you?"

"SUPER!"

Why?

It happened only yesterday. Nancy and I had a restful night, with more sleep than interruptions. As always, I awoke for the sunrise, which was more brilliant than usual. The muted yellows and blending oranges bursting through the window were like an impressionist painting and I considered for a moment whether or not to awaken Nancy.

Nancy had been without a fever for nearly fifteen hours at that point, a blessing that allows her to feel relatively good and lets me worry relatively less. No elevated temperature was a sharp contrast to the day before when she had spiked a temperature of 105 degrees and required more oxygen. The medical team concluded Nancy had pneumonia, and with no innate immunity, the battle seemed stacked against us.

But yesterday morning, even better than the colorful greeting from the rising sun, favorable lab news arrived. Nancy's immune system is making neutrophils. Red cells and platelets, too. Her sleeping bone marrow has awakened at last, and good things are bound to follow.

I attribute this favorable event to your prayers and positive energy.

My deepest heartfelt thanks to each and every one of you.

Summary: The last forty-eight hours have seen a dramatic turnaround in Nancy's condition; her bone marrow is once again generating the specific white blood cells called neutrophils that provide natural immunity and complement the many antibiotics she is taking to fight the pneumonia she has contracted. I've waited anxiously and apprehensively for twenty-eight days to report this spectacular development. If Nancy continues to progress without complications, she will be able to come home in about a week.

SUPER love,

Winnie

Laughter Is the Best Medicine

June 27, 11:34 a.m.

Dear Friends and Family,

Today, Nancy woke up looking bright, more alert, and ready to do something for which I've waited three weeks: have fun. She barely mumbled, "Good morning," before loudly hitting me with the zinger, "Your hair is looking a little ragged, Winnie." Nancy was being kind. (What little hair I still have was more than ragged.)

Disheveled?

Too long?

(Probably both.)

Jayna, who had just arrived to join us, quickly chimed in, "Yeah, Dad, you are having a bad hair day."

I walked over and stood in front of the mirror above the sink on the far wall. I saw a much-too-familiar sight. My hair extended north and south, east and west. All at once.

"All right, Jayna. You can say what you want, but Mom has no room to talk . . . now that she has less hair than me."

Laughter echoed throughout the room, the wonderful sound emanating from both of my girls. Such a sweet sound always warms my heart. The merriment continued for nearly an hour as we chided each other about our dress (or in Nancy's case, the lack of it), our various mannerisms, and even stupid things we'd said years ago—like when I confused Brad Pitt with another actor who had dark hair. Each of our stomachs ached by the time Nancy's chuckling stopped and her eyes closed.

Today, for some unexplained reason, Nancy seems more beautiful than ever before. Her entire bald head seemed shiny this morning—like Charles Barkley.

Last night, I discovered a distinctive mole atop the front right side of Nancy's all too shiny head. Even if her face was hidden, I can now distinguish Nancy's head in a line of a hundred bald heads.

I kissed the newly discovered mole last night and plan to do it several times a day.

And I will cherish each moment.

In fact, I kissed it softly just minutes ago, so as not to awaken Nancy.

Summary: We are learning to have fun again.

Love and laughter
to each of you,

Winnie

No Worries

June 27, 10:39 p.m.

Dear Friends and Family,

As Nancy's strength and activity level have increased, I have a new job: THE WORRY BUSTER.

With important healing to do, there is no issue too small for my attention.

"I forgot to send a present to Enoc, Winnie. He graduated nursing school the week I came to the hospital."

(My beloved deceased grandmother had taught me "a check fits everybody." So a check was in the US Mail within the hour.)

"Winnie, do you remember if I ever talked with Miriam?"

(A much tougher assignment. Nancy hadn't called when a dear friend of ours, Wayne, committed suicide just before Nancy got sick—almost a month ago. Accordingly, I picked up the phone today and called his wife, Miriam, to offer condolences and to tell her about Nancy.)

"Who's feeding the cat, Winnie?"

You guessed it—THE WORRY BUSTER!

It is truly exciting that Nancy is now feeling well enough to focus on other concerns besides making it through the next hour.

Summary: I have a new title—The Worry Buster!

Love and no worries,

Winnie

Anger Isn't a Bad Thing

June 28, 9:46 p.m.

Dear Friends and Family,

After a good day at the office, where staff and patients continue to buoy my spirits, I just arrived at the hospital for my favorite job—Nancy's "nursing assistant's assistant." (And pill holder, ice fetcher, mail reader, bathroom attendant, spirit booster, etc.)

Once again, there are two heads peaking from beneath the new pale-blue covers on Nancy's bed. Both my girls are fast asleep, not even twitching when I burst into the room. I delicately kiss one bald head and one with flowing dirty-blonde tresses before quietly sinking into my bedside chair.

Jayna woke up a minute ago, rubbed her eyes, and smiled at my presence.

"Nice 'doo, Dad," she whispered.

I giggle at her surprise. After all, I'm The Worry Buster! My hair is freshly cut and, at least for one day, is neat and trim. My beard is shorter, too. Anything for my lady.

Minutes later now, Nancy sits up and squints, trying to get me in focus.

"Hi, Winnie. Your hair sure looks good. I like it. You let Stephanie really cut it this time. When did you get here?"

In the last couple of days, as one by one her meds have been discontinued, Nancy has been able to watch TV. But the chemotherapy has affected Nancy's eyesight more than I thought. (My hair hasn't looked good for a decade or more.)

My arrival marks the changing of the "guard."

Jayna has now left to return to her Salt Lake City apartment. A thin slice of normalcy for her? (I can only hope as I ponder how to connect her with friends.)

How do I get her to a movie?

A bar?

Anyplace besides Room 842!

Am I up to making a few calls?

Meanwhile, it is my turn and I am excited for the time alone with my bride.

Our nurse, Denae, has given Nancy her night medicines. Our "other" certified nursing assistant, George, has taken vital signs and won't return for four more hours. The IV bags are full and running. It should be a peaceful time given Nancy's improvement. It's the time of night that Nancy and I typically discuss the future—or potential lack thereof.

Most often, Nancy only speaks about Jaret and Jayna. I speak of Nancy. I cherish this indescribably close time when Nancy is feeling almost normal. For a few precious hours, there will only be the darkness outside, the quiet of our room, and Nancy and me.

Our nurse interrupted our discussion about Jayna; there was one last pill to swallow. But then the magic vanished and, in fact, I got scolded.

"Who said you could offer that candy to the nurses, Winnie? Charlie gave the box of candy to me, not you."

I examine Nancy's beautiful face, incredulous. She's not kidding. Her eyes narrowed and her lower lip extended slightly more than its upper partner. My tears are tempered by a strange realization. Nancy must love me. As far as I know, I'm the only person who experiences her anger. And she needs to have anger.

Summary: We are adjusting to hospital life as best we can.

All our love,

Winnie

A Day Full of Promise

July 2, 10:07 a.m.

Dear Friends and Family,

Today, I rode nonstop to the top of the trail.

Did you know that the multicolored roofs of Park City, when viewed from atop the Lost Prospector mountain bike trail, stretch in all directions? Several rows of gingerbread-like houses, if you've never taken this ride, actually cling to a steep slope below the ridge on the other side of the valley. Almost every day these houses emerge like ghosts from the morning shadows as the rising sun climbs higher in the sky.

Finally.

Generally, I take comfort from the cloudless blue sky, the surrounding scrub oak trees, the late summer yellow sunflowers, and mostly, the solitude. Such exhilarating surroundings always help me gear up for the day's trials. (When I ride my bike, it's my thinking time.)

And new trials are here.

Last night, Nancy developed a new complication.

As usual, she provided the appropriate words: *"I just don't know what to expect, Winnie. Every day is different. And usually, it's awful."* Though she poked me in the stomach as she said this in attempt to make me laugh, I know there is truth in her pronouncement.

I am now fighting the same sentiment.

Despite all my attempts to stay positive for the loved ones around me, once again I am reminded of the obvious.

Life with cancer sucks.

Nancy experienced sharp pain in her left arm yesterday afternoon and evening. Her wrist swelled and her fingers grew tingly. She was forced to remove her simple, gold wedding band when the swelling extended to her fingers. It wasn't a surprise to me when our medical team discovered a blood clot in her right arm, a not uncommon side effect of the special IV line so necessary for her treatment. The team quickly removed the central IV line and Nancy was immediately started on blood thinners.

Medically, this is a tough setback. But psychologically, the setback is even worse. Nancy's highly anticipated hospital departure has been postponed.

Just minutes ago, I received the call.

Today, will mark the end of Chapter 1 in *Adventures in Cancer Land*. Despite the blood clot discovered yesterday, Nancy will return to Woodland today!

Since Nancy will be coming to Woodland on oxygen, she won't be venturing to our upstairs family room, the place we normally hang out. Our downstairs living room, consciously devoid of furniture since we moved in twenty-one years ago because of its' natural beauty (a large hand-placed stone fireplace; a twenty-four-foot wood ceiling; and floor-to-ceiling windows with a pristine view of the river, trees, and mountains), now includes a long couch for napping, a coffee table big enough to embrace two full meals, and several comfy chairs including a recliner. The room's floor-to-ceiling windows face south, allowing brilliant sunshine to fill the room from early morning to late afternoon. (We hope the contrast with our one, tiny hospital window and artificially lit hospital room will warm Nancy's heart and strengthen her frail body.)

Though our newly furnished living room should be ideal, we anticipate that Nancy will spend most of her time in our bedroom. After all, Nancy's mission at home is to rest and regain her strength for the next round of chemo. She will be greeted by a brand new, ultracomfortable king-size foam bed adorned with soft sheets, down pillows, and a new down comforter featuring a deep-red paisley design.

Our ground floor bedroom, like the newly appointed living room, opens to a deck whose entire far edge is flower boxes that contain multicolored pansies, daisies, and other varieties of wild flowers. The deck overlooks the Provo River as it winds through the property, the far side lined with cottonwood trees, aspen trees, and scrub oak.

Bells and buzzers will now be replaced by the melodic sounds of birds and bugs. The smells of summer in the country will replace the antiseptic smell of the hospital.

Home.

A great place for healing.

Summary: Nancy leaves Room 842 today after thirty-five days. We are returning home!

Love,

Winnie

A Day of Less Promise

July 2, 2:10 p.m.

Dear Friends and Family,

To say I'm a bit excited about Nancy's return home would be like saying I am a bit hungry after eating no food for an entire month.

My mind is overflowing with details. I've picked up about sixty feet of remote oxygen tubing so Nancy can walk through the house without pulling a canister of oxygen.

I've stockpiled dressing supplies, sterile gloves, needles, and the like.

I've checked and rechecked Nancy's medicines, ensuring we have enough pills for her seventeen days at home.

There is still food to buy, cleaning to do, and calls to make. My list is long but not begrudged. I want this to be a singularly special time.

While relating so many of our day-to-day stories, I've omitted some medical details.

So it's time to catch up.

Nancy's blood status has improved dramatically. Her hematocrit, a test that measures the number of oxygen-carrying red blood cells, was so low she required transfusions every few days following the chemotherapy. That particular test is now normal.

Platelets, the particles that stop bleeding, were also low for most of this hospitalization. Nancy received platelet transfusions even more frequently than the red blood cells. Over the last week, her platelets have rocketed into the normal range. She's allowed to blow her nose again. (The simple pleasures of life.)

Most importantly, Nancy's infection-fighting white blood cells have finally rebounded. Her total white cell count is now at the same level as yours and mine. She no longer needs to wear a mask when she walks the hall on the eighth floor and will soon leave her artificially sterile world. (I'm probably allowed to kiss her on the lips, though it will feel strange. Which one of us will be more scared?)

Just nine days ago, Nancy had a fever to 105 degrees and rapidly developing pneumonia. Though nothing grew on the almost daily cultures, the infectious disease specialists suspected a fungus named Aspergillum. But the doctors were uncertain.

Uncertainty.

Uncertainty is part of our daily lives. We try to banish it to a remote corner of our brains. We try to exile it from our souls. Still it is always lurking.

At present, there are unwanted spots on Nancy's chest X-ray, reflecting a remaining, uncertain dark force. We will complete the battle at home; Nancy will leave the hospital in remission from the leukemia, but still on oxygen and an antifungal medicine.

On an early morning bike ride a few days ago, I ran into a friend and female patient atop a mountain overlooking Park City. I was exhilarated to see the sun quickly ascending up over the horizon and she inhaled deeply and said, "Today is a new day, full of promise," before waving and running off.

Her words echo my feelings today.

Nancy is coming home to rest and prepare for round two. But there is more to think about than the next round. Two days ago, we sat down with one of our oncologists, Dr. Elizabeth Prystas. "The High Priestess," as Nancy has nicknamed her since the pronunciation is the same, took her customary seat next to Nancy's bed. Though slight in build, Dr. Prystas has an unusually commanding presence.

"All of your numbers look good, Nancy. The pulmonary people tell me your lungs are improving rapidly. The infectious disease folks have you down to taking only one drug. Let's plan on going home the day after tomorrow."

"What happens next?" Nancy's voice was steady, and her mind seemed clear. (A few days ago, she would have fallen asleep in the middle of a question.)

"Let's see, we'll plan on you coming back for the next phase of treatment in two weeks. No, since you'll be leaving on a Friday, we'll start again on a Monday. That'll make it seventeen days.

"When you come back, we'll start the treatment phase we call consolidation. Though you're in remission now, experience tells us that if we don't give you more chemotherapy, you will relapse. So we will plan on four rounds of consolidation."

I can read Nancy's face pretty well after more than a quarter century. There was disappointment in her eyes. Both of us thought there were only three more hospital stays. (Didn't "Captain" Morton, the High Priestess's partner tell us that?) Nancy coughed and turned away. When she turned back, her face was calm and composed.

"And what about a bone marrow transplant? Do we talk about that now?"

"Good question, Nancy. We'll want you and Winnie to meet with the bone marrow team during your two-week holiday. Probably near the end of that time period, after you've gained strength and perspective. A transplant procedure is very difficult. Our decision will be when to do it. Though you've shown great resilience and toughness, we have to decide if we should consider a transplant early, after the first consolidation treatment. Or if we should save it as a rescue procedure—if the other treatments don't work."

"What would you do, Dr. Prystas?"

I was dumbfounded by this question. Until today, Nancy had not wanted information beyond the near horizon. With some real lows recently, I had worried about Nancy's resolve.

But now?

Nancy was stepping up to the plate and swinging for the big picture.

The High Priestess has short, black hair that surrounds a soft, kind face. Her dark-blue eyes overflow with compassion. She speaks in a voice that could say, *"Your son is going to Iraq,"* and you'd think it was all right. But I almost fell off my chair when Dr. Prystas responded, "Your leukemia seems to be a good one, treatmentwise. Personally, I would do the four consolidation courses and hope you are in the 15–20% that get cured."

My face flushed with blood—15–20%?

How can the survival rates keep changing?

At one time, the "Captain" told us "almost 50%."

Another time it was 30–40%. I even wrote those numbers down.

Once again, I fought back against the moisture behind my contacts.

Dr. Prystas continued: "I'd wait and see. I would save the transplant in case the leukemia returns."

Unlike me, Nancy's expression was serene. Unlike me, she was ready. When I squeezed her hand, she squeezed back. More tightly.

Summary: Nancy' blood work is reflecting a positive reality. It is a new day, full of promise—but a little less than yesterday.

With much love,

Winnie

Singing in the Sunlight

July 2, 12:23 p.m.

Dear Friends and Family,

Since I am at work, I have to write quickly. It is hard to type because my mind is racing a bit too fast for my hands. Additionally, my hands are uncontrollably shaking with excitement.

Jayna just called. There were no surprises at the hospital this morning and Nancy is in the car beside her. The back seat of the car and trunk are filled to the brim with room decorations because Jayna arranged the car so that Nancy can recline (and sleep) if she wants to or has the need to rest.

So far, all Nancy wants to do is feel the warm sunshine on her skin, comment on the buildings and flowers and people, and roll down the window so the wind can blow on her face. She wants to smell the fresh scent of summer flowers from the fields on either side of the highway ascending the canyon leading home, too. She and Jayna are singing along with the radio, and Jayna tells me Nancy is dancing in her seat.

I am sad not to be with them now and even sadder that I won't be there when Nancy walks into our bedroom. But I can see in my mind's eye the look on her face when she first sees our new bed. (Thirty-five days must have been an eternity for Nancy to be confined to her rather small hospital room.)

My shift ends early so I will be home for dinner. As has occurred each and every day since Nancy was hospitalized, a friend and supporter has provided dinner. Nancy has so many friends. I have witnessed and been the recipient of more kindness this past month than I ever expected in ten lifetimes. (Tonight's meal includes rib eye steak—Nancy's favorite and one containing lots of protein and iron. Thanks, Joannie!)

A few answers to questions you have recently sent me:

(1) Nancy is now able to have "live" flowers, and if you want to send a card during the next seventeen glorious days, use our home (Woodland) address.

(2) When I ask Nancy what she wants to do, at the top of her list is reading your (already received) best wishes, letters, and emails. My feeble attempt to read a paragraph here and there before her slumber each night has been inadequate, and I look forward to rereading them to or with her.

(3) Should you call Nancy? This is a tough one because I really don't know the answer. My plan is this: feel free to call our home phone. There will be a phone in our bedroom, where I expect Nancy will spend most of her initial days; it will be unplugged unless she chooses otherwise. We may or may not answer in one of the other rooms depending on what we are doing. Even if we don't answer, there is an answering machine, and I know she will enjoy listening to any message you leave. I suspect at some point Nancy will have enough extra strength to converse. Right now, she plans on putting her total energy into preparations for the next round of chemotherapy.

(4) I will address your requests for potential visits as soon as I have a better understanding of this new phase.

As usual, dial or write with any questions or thoughts. My mobile phone won't work when I am in Woodland, because the electrons don't reach that far for "technological" reasons that for some reason are beyond my comprehension.

Summary: Finally, today is the day Nancy leaves the hospital and returns home.

All my love,

Winnie

Christmas in July

July 9, 8:08 p.m.

Dear Friends and Family,

For the past twenty years or so, I've sent our Christmas greetings well after the holidays. Most often, our cards have not made it to the post office until the end of spring or in early summer. I am embarrassed to admit that one year I barely mailed them before the first snowfall.

In my defense, I was loosely following the precedent from my many years of running the Old Faithful Clinic in Yellowstone National Park. Almost every year there, the first snowflakes arrive in late August coinciding with the end of the summer season when employees return to home, college, or their next adventure.

Many decades ago, two feet of snow blanketed the park on August 25, so a large group of employees pretended it was Christmas. They wore makeshift reindeer costumes to their jobs, sang yuletide songs, and drank eggnog.

A tradition was born.

Since then, Yellowstone employees "celebrate" Christmas every August 25. They call it "Christmas in summer" and the tourists love it.

With the final week of December being the busiest tourist week in Park City every year, I loosely adopted Yellowstone's tradition. Annually, I wait until the holiday bug bites me sometime after ski season. It might be May or it might be late August. I never know when I will be seized by the moment. It doesn't matter. One day when I feel like summarizing my year for our friends and family, I declare it my holiday season. I toast to Santa and out go my cards.

Not this year.

Yesterday, on July 8, there were nine people sitting around our dining room table and Julie, Nancy's longtime friend from Tucson, asked, "Your Christmas tree is really beautiful. How long has it been up?" Our dining room is two steps above the living room and looks out over the sitting area below. At the far edge of the living room, a fourteen-foot highly decorated Christmas tree resplendently resides.

"Well," I answered, "About ten years."

"It's been eleven, Dadder," Jayna interjected. "It's Christmas all year at our house, Julie." There was general laughter as I explained Christmas in Yellowstone and my long personal practice of choosing the exact day on my whim, and how having a Christmas tree up year round made that possible.

Jaret was too excited to let this conversation continue. "Happy Birthday, Mom!" he announced as he handed Nancy a present and kissed her on the cheek.

Our birthday dinner group was the largest Nancy has hosted since she fell ill. In addition to Jaret, Jayna, me, and Nancy's sister, Linda, Jayna's college "parents," Howard and Rhonda, who are visiting their son Louis in Denver from New York, also flew over for the occasion. Louis has been one of Jayna's best friends in college and his family "adopted" Jayna for several holidays when she couldn't make it back to Utah. All of these guests were expected (and preapproved) by Nancy. Julie, Nancy's first flying partner at TWA, was a notable and truly unexpected surprise. Nancy's face lit up when she rang the doorbell; she hadn't seen Julie in years.

For me, a full house of guests echoed times past, and Nancy embraced the happiness of being surrounded by a jovial group with one common goal: to have this be Nancy's best birthday ever. Julie prepared a mouth-watering meal of baked fish and tempura vegetables and matched it with her favorite sake. Nancy gave it her highest praise: "This tastes better than the hospital pancakes." To complement the meal, Howard and Rhonda related their recent adventures in Japan. Though all the serving dishes were empty by meal's end, our biggest (and very tiring) activity yesterday was laughing. (Quite honestly, I had to make an excuse and leave the table twice because the carefree mood provoked tears I didn't want Nancy or the others to see.)

When the birthday cake's arrival was imminent, each of us donned a brightly colored, cone-shaped party hat. Mine was blue and had orange balloons on it; the elastic band that held it in place made my beard tuck under my neck. I am sure I looked more ridiculous than usual even though the hat hid my bald spot as it stood straight up on the back of my head. Nancy's bonnet was pink with blue and white balloons. She looked both natural and elegant even though the twenty-five-cent cardboard hat only partially covered her beautiful and completely hairless head. The cap matched her new pink scarf and exquisitely highlighted her skin tone and eye color.

I must admit—when she had modeled the scarf for me earlier in the day before our guests arrived, she had enthusiastically asserted, "I don't have to wear a hospital gown tonight!" An ear-to-ear smile spanned Nancy's face. Her eyes sparkled in the early evening sunlight. I froze the moment in my mind's camera. It was our happiest snapshot in a long time.

Nancy's requested cake was chocolate decadence. I put five candles on one edge and seven on the other to mark fifty-seven years. I didn't light them. Nancy still has a cannula in her nose delivering oxygen, so no flames are allowed in the house. But that didn't dampen Nancy's spirit. Without a second's hesitation, she pretended to blow out each and every candle one by one. We cheered and sang "Happy Birthday" again and again. There were more stories. There was more laughter. I didn't tuck Nancy into bed until almost eleven.

July 8 was truly a special day this year. Our family had dreamed of this birthday yet wondered if we'd be celebrating.

For me, July 8 was also Christmas.

The best one ever.

Summary: July 8 finds our family hosting a real party. Friends and family surrounded Nancy for her fifty-eighth birthday. It was such a wonderful celebration that we also celebrated the day as Christmas.

Very much love,

Winnie

A Trip to Normal

July 14, 6:08 a.m.

Dear Friends and Family,

Once again, our new bright-red paisley comforter has swallowed Nancy's body. Only a familiar cute bald head peaks from beneath its left upper edge. As I regard her shiny head, it strikes me that I can hardly remember what Nancy looks like with hair.

Not surprisingly, I used to think that no hair was undesirable. Not now.

Nancy senses my gaze, slowly opens her eyes, and smiles back at me. Instinctively, I rub the growing fuzz and gently kiss the special mole just like I do every morning and every evening. This action has become our new ritual.

One has to find positives when dealing with cancer.

"Good morning, beautiful." I whisper in Nancy's ear after placing a second kiss on her right earlobe.

"I'm not beautiful, am I?"

There is no need for me to answer.

Today is a very big day.

Today we will venture to Salt Lake City.

Today we visit her oncologist.

Instead of asking if Nancy wants breakfast in bed, I urge her to sit and then stand up. She has only left our property three times in the nearly two weeks we've been home. The first time was for a chest X-ray at my Park City office to confirm that her pneumonia had disappeared. Another time Nancy announced, "I feel really strong today. Let's go to the market." (I've never enjoyed the Kamas grocery store more.) And then yesterday, we actually walked to the Woodland Cash Store at the end of our block. Nancy is light years stronger now than when she arrived home.

But today is distinctly different; Nancy is feeling strong and better.

"What do you think of this hat with my outfit, Winnie?"

As we prepare for our trip, she has changed clothes at least five times.

"They look really good together to me, my love."

Nancy knows that asking me "Which color goes best?" or "Which shirt is most flattering?" is like asking me to translate Chinese. Ignoring my words, she sighs, and turns to her trusted counselor Jayna, who has just joined us. Minutes later, they have chosen an outfit that is a perfect match. Both the pants suit and hat highlight her eyes. That, even I can see.

Although Nancy was so excited she "raced" me to the car for the hour's ride to Salt Lake City, we rode in silence for at least ten minutes as I watched her soak in the scenery outside the window. When she coughed, I broke the silence: "How you doing, darlin'?" I'd stolen the line from the movie *The Big Easy* and gave a southern flare to the word 'darling.'

Nancy didn't answer immediately, and I wondered if something was wrong. Then with as loud a voice as I've heard in a month and a half, I was startled by her shout.

"I feel free!"

Nancy is genuinely and deeply happy.

At last she is "unhooked."

No hospital bracelets.

No IVs.

And today, no oxygen tube is in her nose.

After twelve days at home, Nancy is as normal as she can be. Only someone who has had needles in both arms, tubes in unmentionable places, and a mask over her face for days on end can know the joy I see next to me. Nancy's eyes shine like turquoise jewels.

The hour's trip goes all too quickly. Too soon, Nancy returns to medicine's clutches.

"You're going to feel a little sting, followed by a burn. Here's the sting."

Nancy lies on an exam table next to my chair. On the oppo-site side is Dr. Morton. To me, Dr. Russ Morton is the "attend-ing physician," the doctor ultimately in charge of Nancy's case. But to my girls, he is "Captain," the leader of our platoon. Nancy is holding my hand and I don't want to let go. Her bone marrow procedure is about to begin.

The bone marrow is the womb of all blood components. It is where any recurrence of Nancy's leukemia will first be detected. My free hand is sweaty. I don't snap my fingers on that hand either. I am too busy repeating the same words silently that are echoing in my head. *Please, bone marrow—be all right.*

I watch Dr. Morton skillfully inject Nancy's back. "Here's the burn," he warns.

Nancy is an amazing trooper. When suturing a patient's lacerations, as I do on most workdays, I administer the same numbing medicine. I often hear a loud scream or words I can't repeat in this note. I see loved ones' hands nearly broken during a moment similar to the one I am in now. Nancy's hand squeeze, however, is barely perceptible.

Captain picks up a very large syringe attached to a huge needle. He is about to bore into Nancy's hip, the best place to extract the precious marrow.

"You may feel this a touch."

The sound of crushing bone fills the room inescapably. My hand feels another tiny squeeze. Nancy amazes me again. Her facial expression is serene. When Dr. Morton announces that the test is finished, Nancy smiles and says, "Thank you, Dr. Morton."

I don't belabor the significance of the bone marrow test to Nancy. In fact, I barely mention it on the way home except to ask if her hip is sore. She replies, "A little," and contin-ues to be mesmerized by the scenery as we head back up Parley's Canyon toward Park City and Woodland.

Captain is a low-key guy. His words didn't alert Nancy to the bone marrow test's importance. But I know too much. Sometimes I wish I were a park ranger or working in a gas sta-tion. I am still struggling as we prepare for our second round of chemotherapy.

How much do I ask?

How much do I read?

How much research should I do?

And the worst: How much medical information do I tell Nancy, Jaret, or Jayna?

I want our last five days at home to be worry free. I still fancy myself as "The Worry Buster!" But the next day, as I dial the oncologists' office, I have a lonely and frightened feeling.

"Drs. Morton and Prystas' office."

"Yes . . . this is Nancy Winn's husband, Winnie. Dr. Morton said I could call today to find out my wife's bone marrow test results from yesterday."

"Dr. Winn, let me check for you. Dr. Morton did tell me you'd be calling."

Thirty seconds of silence seems like an eternity.

"I'm sorry, but the test results are not back yet, Dr. Winn. For some reason the lab is a little slow today. May I call you when we get them?"

Many answers roll through my head. I choose a socially acceptable one.

"Yes, that'd be great. Thanks."

I hurry back to my patients, reminding myself that I am working today and they deserve my full attention. I do look at my mobile phone periodically to be sure I have power, that the vibrate mode is working, and that I haven't mysteriously missed a call.

Finally, I feel a familiar buzz in my chest pocket. The caller ID reads LDS Hospital. I scurry to an empty room, feeling blood rush to my temples.

"Winnie, Russ Morton here. I've got good news. . . ."

Summary: Nancy's bone marrow test is normal. At present, she is leukemia free.

Much love,

Winnie

I Yam What I Yam

July 18, 3:01 a.m.

Dear Friends and Family,

Nancy and I have always enjoyed and made the most of her airline's employee travel benefits. Free travel has allowed us frequent family trips back east and made exotic beaches and wild jungles accessible. Historic sites and captivating museums have often been our "destinations" as we've ventured to various world nooks and crannies. Still, when I reflect on every trip we've ever taken, one thing remains constant: I'm never sad to return home.

Why?

Nancy and I are privileged to live in an exceptional locale—Park City, Utah. We have great friends nearby, majestic mountains in all directions, and four distinct seasons. Whether for skiing in winter or hiking and biking in summer, we live in a "destination" resort. People from the far reaches of this country and the far corners of the world come to our "neck of the woods" to spend their holidays.

Today, our "home" vacation ends.

And this time, I don't want our retreat to be over.

Despite my misgivings, tomorrow we return to the "penthouse" at LDS Hospital for Nancy's next round of chemotherapy. Room 844. We anticipate being there a full month. Our newest hospital address will be Nancy Winn, C/O LDS Hospital, 8th Avenue and C Street, Salt Lake City, Utah 84143. As before, Nancy's white cells will come to be extinct. Only sterile plastic flowers will adorn her room, 844.

Nancy's body and spirit are recharged.

Was it the soothing sounds of our real home?

Or the gurgling river?

Or the sweet smell of fresh flowers?

Or maybe it was the chirping birds?

Quite simply, there is no adjective worthy of Nancy's facial expressions as she re-experienced the taste of home-cooked meals. (Again, many thanks to our "local" friends for the daily presents left anonymously on our doorstep.) So many "home" aspects have contributed to Nancy's recuperation. Her mind is clear again and her spirit is back. The last seventeen days, we've laughed a lot and cried just a little.

In many ways, our previous hospitalization is a fog for Nancy. Much of it bypassed her memory bank, a condition that is quite fortunate. Since coming home, Nancy has discovered the one part of our last hospital stay I didn't want her to miss—the many people who have cared about her and sent their love. When she first came to Woodland, I placed a huge stack of cards on the night table beside her. Today, as we prepare to leave, the stack has disappeared, now filed in a very special drawer.

Though I remain "in charge" of Nancy's correspondence and sometimes have to read to her, during the past two weeks, Nancy has eagerly devoured your emails and letters. The effect has been crucial. Nancy's mood has been lifted by the unwavering support you have "beamed" in her direction. She exhibits new resolve and is ready for tomorrow. Actually, more so than me. (I'd rather our present vacation extend indefinitely.)

Jaret and Jayna have also cherished the relative normalcy of the last two weeks. It has been a much-needed quiet period and a well-deserved intimate time for our family. Like Nancy, they seem ready—at least outwardly.

So we return to the hospital tomorrow with a clean slate. There is no leukemia detectable in Nancy's body.

Before bed last night, Nancy flexed her biceps and flashed her arm muscles like Popeye (without either the pipe or can of spinach) and quipped, "I'm ready."

I'm also ready to hold Nancy's hand and absorb any and every squeeze.

And we're both comforted that each of you is part of our team.

Thanks.

Summary: We return to the hospital tomorrow with Nancy focusing on the future—while tugging me in that direction, too.

Fondly,

Winnie

A Tip of the Hat to Chemotherapy

July 25, 6:15 a.m.

Dear Friends and Family,

I am feeling silly today. (Perhaps giddy would be a more appropriate description.) My hands are linked behind my head and my feet are up on a stool. I am watching my bride sleep as if she is floating on a cloud. Even though we are still in the hospital, for once I feel relaxed. There is no hint of pain on Nancy's expressionless face.

Unlike many other times, I also detect no worry. As I look more closely, Nancy's beautiful bald head sports several brave strands of hair. I have to suppress a laugh. The little hairs randomly dot her scalp, standing straight and tall like telephone poles. They seem to whisper to me, "Look. I'm back already."

The early morning light is uneven, and even as I sneak close to her, I can't distinguish the color of the new growth. (We do have the same great, albeit tiny, view of the mountains through our window in Room 844. Today, however, clouds mostly obscure the sunrise.) Though I'm eager to know if Nancy's hair will return as blonde, red, white (or even blue, I don't care), it may be many months before we know the answer. Nancy has just completed her second round of chemotherapy. The new, cute hair strands will soon adorn her pillow, leaving her head bright and shiny again.

I've been pondering how to better explain Nancy's medical treatment. Having watched more TV these past months than in entire previous years, I'll utilize that medium. Pretend you are sitting with me and we are watching TV. A commercial for

119

Nancy's major chemotherapy drug, AraC, interrupts our game show, sitcom, or sporting event.

"Take AraC and watch the 'bad guy' leukemia cells melt away from the bone marrow," a soothing TV pitch woman begins.

On the screen, the image of a cave emerges. There are stalactites and stalagmites in every direction. However, this cave looks different from any that you and I have seen before. The cave is fluorescent pink. The brightness almost hurts our eyes. The caption below the cave entrance reads "Inside Nancy's Bone Marrow."

As the camera pans the cave, we notice that there are black spots on the walls. The camera zooms in on one of the spots and what is revealed is startling. Each black spot is an ugly, gnome-like creature with a twisted, wrinkled body and a horrid face sporting a nefarious smile. The creature's eyes protrude on stalks from its face and are huge and bloodshot. The shifting pupils stare at us eerily as if searching for prey.

The new caption on the screen is a single word: LEUKEMIA.

Suddenly, a brilliant gold-colored gas flows through the pink cave. One by one, the dark creatures fall from their perches on the walls, vaporized in a puff of gray smoke. When the gold gas disappears from the picture, the bone marrow is transformed. In just seconds, it has become a deep (and healthy) red.

The soothing TV voice continues: *"In three times out of ten, AraC will eradicate the leukemia cells. Just like Drano ridding scum from your toilet's pipes."*

The scene changes. Now on the TV is a swing set resting amid a field of knee-high, bright-yellow sunflowers. As we get closer, we see a little boy being pushed higher and higher by his mother. A close-up of the boy and his mother show matching freckled faces and award-winning smiles. As the mother turns away from the camera, she removes her long, flowing blonde ringlets that are revealed to be a wig. The boy's eyes widen in surprise at his mother's lack of hair, but he gently touches her fuzzy head with one finger, then two. The little boy eagerly rubs his mother's head with both of his tiny hands. They both laugh. The boy kisses his mother's cheek.

The soothing voice continues in the background during this scene: *"Of course, AraC is not for everybody. Occasionally . . . well, actually often, there are significant side effects. The most common side effects are vomiting, diarrhea, headaches, and painful skin rashes. Please call your doctor if your kidneys fail, you have brain damage, or die. Actually, if you die, have someone else call because it would be a very long-distance call and our toll-free number might not work. You should not take AraC if you do not have leukemia. In fact, you probably should discuss taking this medicine with your doctor even if you do have leukemia. AraC is a dangerous drug."*

Once the commercial is over, you are back to watching Jeopardy or some other "entertainment" diversion. (Me? I'd be shaking in my chair, worrying about AraC's potential problems.)

We just imagined the ALL-LEUKEMIA channel. The cave part of the "commercial" is a technique I mentioned previously in my letters called visualization. Nancy and I use it with each of her chemotherapy treatments. She sometimes falls asleep. When I visualize, I either laugh or cry when I'm finished.

Nancy has just awakened me from my Walter Mitty–like revelry: "Winnie, what are you doing up so early? I hoped you would sleep late today. Didn't you have only four hours the night before last when you were on call? And maybe just five last night?"

I jump from my chair, move to Nancy's bed, and place a loud kiss on my favorite mole atop her shiny head.

"You are right, my love. But I feel great. Look at your IV bag? Not only did you sleep all night, you're less than an hour away from finishing this round of chemotherapy drugs. And you've had no side effects."

Nancy and I look at each other without speaking.

Six doses of AraC are fading into the rearview mirror. Nancy and I were plenty nervous when her initial bag was hung six days ago. I had flashbacks to the first day of her first round of chemotherapy when she entered the hospital, when Nancy's lungs filled with fluid and she required more oxygen by the minute. There was scary talk about the ICU and a respirator. I remember wondering if Nancy would survive that first day.

Chemotherapy drugs, though lifesaving, are dangerous. Unbelievably dangerous. Just like in my made-up commercial. And even though Nancy has only received the same drug at the same dosage for the same amount of days, this round is different. A new Nancy has returned to the battle this time.

Strong.

Confident.

Ready.

And with Popeye muscles.

For us, AraC is Nancy's Vitamin C—her special orange juice. Despite the negative risks, Nancy has now made it through six doses without a hitch. In fact, she has actually watched DVD's (and Jeopardy) and eaten like she was still on vacation at home. (Well, not exactly. The food is nowhere as delicious as the gourmet meals provided by our local friends.) Yesterday, we even did twelve laps up and down the hall in a single outing. During Nancy's first hospitalization, three laps was her personal best.

Today, I write this letter with a smile stretched all the way across my face. Nancy's smile is similar, too. We know that it's just a single day among a long line of difficult days to come, but we will enjoy every last feel-good minute.

Why?

AraC's expected and desired effects will increase dramatically over the next several days. Nancy will, like last time, become severely neutropenic with no white cells to fight infections. Already, this morning, she has been asked to wear a mask for her walks in the hall. Her platelets will drop critically low, necessitating replacement platelets every few days to avoid serious bleeding. Her oxygen-carrying red blood cells will continue to decrease, and soon Nancy will require transfusions again.

The result?

Nancy will once again be at high risk for fevers as unusual germs attack her body. She will have to be careful to avoid bumps and the resultant bleeding. She will be physically weakened due to the coming anemia.

And yes, sadly, she will once again feel just plain crappy.

Our arsenal is full, however. We have ever-increasing experience. Nancy's scary first month of treatment, called induction, is now just a vague memory. She still has no sign of recurrence, so she is technically in remission. When the final red drop of AraC enters her veins, we'll have made it through the first round of consolidation chemotherapy. It's called "consolidation" because the new chemo helps "consolidate" our gains against the cancer. If she can make it through this next rough period, we will be able to go home for another two-week vacation.

"Let me get that for you, sweetie," I say as I see her reaching for the book on the far end of the nightstand. Nancy ignores me. She sits up, stretches an arm, and retrieves the other book she is reading, the thriller *The Lions of Lucerne* by Brad Thor, a friend of ours.

"I can do it, Winnie. I should do everything I can while I still feel so good."

Yes, Nancy does feel good and I am giddy.

On the phone last night, she described recent events to a childhood friend. It was the first time she had called someone other than family.

"You know, except for this awful disease, it has been a really positive experience. I've learned a whole lot of people care about me . . ."

Critically, Nancy is basking in the warmth of your love and support.

And I can think of nothing more important in helping with her fight.

Thanks so much from the bottom of our hearts.

Summary: This morning on day seven of hospitalization two, Nancy is finishing her chemotherapy, having tolerated it well. Though she feels great now, we know she will get sick again as the medicine attacks her and her leukemia.

All our love,

Winnie

Parting Is Such Sweet Sorrow

July 28, 1:40 p.m.

Dear Friends and Family,

Today is a very sad day in our "penthouse" hospital room. *Why?*
(It's not what you think.)
August 1 is "back to school" day for Nancy's sister, Linda. Tomorrow she will be preparing schedules and attending workshops. Lesson plans and seating charts will replace hospital sleepovers and time spent with her nephew, Jaret. Linda will board a plane and travel 1,787 miles east to Dalton, Georgia, where she teaches middle school students ESL (English as a second language).

For the past six weeks, Linda has been the most amazing sister-in-law. Plunging into our family chaos, she immediately made an impact. She substituted for her sister, Nancy, helping Jaret successfully finish his junior year of college. Linda ensured that Jayna always had at least one friend for movies. (During this time period, Jayna had difficulty being around anyone outside our family circle.) Linda even made sure I remained grounded so I could lead my "double life" as a doctor in Park City and as a husband (and caretaker) in Salt Lake City. Simply put, if I looked up the word "godsend" in the dictionary, I am certain I'd find a picture of Linda.

But even more important than what Linda provided for us (Jaret, Jayna, and me) is what she has provided for Nancy—a link to her normal past life before leukemia. And as Linda was preparing to leave for the airport yesterday, it was no different from what I had witnessed for many weeks.

"Oh, one more thing, Nancy," Linda said. "I guess we don't need those towels I bought for the guest room in Woodland. We found the missing ones."

"Not a problem, Linda. I can take them back for you."

As Nancy took a sip of water, her eyes shined brightly and she sat straight up in her hospital bed. True, she had no hair. Yes, she was dressed in a less-than-fashionable blue polka dot hospital gown. And if you were to make a close examination of either arm you would observe the telltale bruises. But if I had closed my eyes I would have sworn that Nancy's speech and delivery would have found her sipping that glass of water in a restaurant or in our home. Nancy sounded and acted completely normal.

Does she really have leukemia?

Is she really fighting a life-threatening disease?

In all honesty, my slight chuckle disguised the feeling of moistness behind my contacts.

"What a great idea, Nancy! Will you take your three IV bags with you? Wear your mask? Which hat would you like?"

Linda has a unique and unusual laugh that starts out low in pitch and volume, includes some intermediate breaths while winding up, and then finishes with a loud, midrange cackle that crescendos to a high note bordering on a near scream. A distinctive noise combination that would be recognizable from the other side of a football stadium, her laugh can in a flash fill every inch of our hospital room. And like a yawn, Linda's laugh is contagious.

The significance of Nancy's remark was not lost amid our laughter. Nine days into hospitalization two, after six maximum doses of the chemotherapy drug AraC, with her red blood cell count low enough to require transfusions, her white blood cells absent, and her blood clotting platelet cells in the "basement," Nancy felt good enough to contemplate running up to the outlet mall to return towels for her sister.

I flashed back to Nancy's declaration last night before she went to sleep.

"Winnie, sometimes I feel almost normal."

Nancy is a true trooper, and at least this time, we have been lucky. This hospitalization has been less traumatic than we anticipated. She is walking the halls, eating everything in sight, and best of all, laughing a lot. And her demeanor has not gone unnoticed by the nursing staff.

Our primary nurse this week, Anne, told me the other day, "Winnie, your wife is amazing. We've never seen someone exercise like she does when her bone marrow is totally shut down."

And I don't believe that I've mentioned this observation in prior notes, but more than once I've had staff members give variations of what our certified nursing assistant told me last week, "Winnie, your wife is my favorite patient. Ever." (Will has worked on the bone marrow floor for seven years.)

Mine too, Will.

As Linda stood up to get ready to depart for the airport, she gave her sister a final hug but not a kiss. Kissing spreads germs, and Nancy has no infection-fighting white cells left in her blood. (Should I tell Jayna about kissing and germs?)

Over the past six weeks, I've witnessed incredible closeness and caring between two sisters. (I can only hope that Jaret and Jayna will be so connected.) During the last hug between Nancy and Linda, I felt like a voyeur. Though the sisters talk "southern" and avoid direct discussion about most things, including their closeness, their tender bond warms me to the center of my soul.

As Linda and I walked to the elevator, we did share some "germs" as I held her a last time. In all candor, partings have always been a mystery to me—especially now. I think to myself, "When will I see you again, Linda? Where will Nancy be?"—and the question I try not to ponder, "How will Nancy be doing?"

When I returned, my bride was in tears. We held hands in silence. Then Nancy dropped my hand, and I heard a deep sigh. The melancholy painted across her face was replaced by a smile—the one that makes me melt like chocolate in the warm summer sun.

"This isn't really that bad, Winnie. The people who work here are so nice. I don't have to cook or clean. I can read as many books as I want. And I get to spend so much time with my family."

She grabbed my hand again, and I noticed a playful twinkle in her eyes. "You know, Winnie, except for this disease, it's almost fun."

Of course, Nancy left out the pokes and prods, the sleep interruptions, and, of course, the uncertainty of our future. I do so marvel at her spirit. She's already adjusted to Linda's departure and the void she leaves behind before I can even take a deep breath.

Summary: Nancy's sister returned to Georgia today and she will be sorely missed.

Very much love,

Winnie

Donuts and the Nadir

July 28, 8:40 p.m.

Dear Friends and Family,

Linda's departure was more draining than Nancy will admit. She didn't fall asleep midsentence, but she did take a nap shortly after Linda left and didn't awaken for three hours. When she finally sat up in bed, a classic impish expression returned to her face. Nancy's sky-blues looked up and away, a little wrinkle toward the tip of her nose appeared and her playful voice gave me my marching orders.

Pointing toward the door, she commanded, "Yes, I'd like another donut. I get to eat anything I want." Obediently, I raced down the nine floors of steps, two at a time, and then raced back up, too. Nancy literally inhaled both a classic glazed and a chocolate cream-filled donut. She finished both before I could take my last bite of my sugar-covered jelly donut.

I could watch Nancy eat donuts all day.

But as is often the case, the roller coaster called leukemia turned downward today, just when we were beginning to feel more positive and comfortable. Dr. Prystas stopped by unexpectedly for a quick report.

"Nancy, the tests have come back on both your brother and sister. Unfortunately, neither of them is a match. We'll set up a conference call with the bone marrow experts as soon as possible to explain the implications and discuss what are our next steps."

As you might imagine, Nancy and I were disappointed and attempted to play cards to distract us. Not far into the game, Nancy was dealing the cards and told me, "You know, Winnie, my PIC line is a little tender." (The PIC line is a very special IV that enters a large vein from Nancy's chest and makes all her treatments easier since it is a large needle capable of allowing lots of fluid to pass through it in a small amount of time. Additionally, it only infrequently has to be changed and does not tie up one of her arms as normal IVs do.)

When Nancy's discomfort was explored further by the medical team this afternoon, a blood clot was discovered and the IV had to be pulled and blood thinners started immediately. To make matters worse, Nancy appears to have developed a localized infection called cellulitis at the PIC line entry site. (With Nancy's immunity at its lowest point, not having a good IV and needing potent antibiotics to fight the infection is not a favorable combination.)

We're scared. But Nancy remains upbeat and positive. And we did catch both the clot and infection early.

Summary: Even with the maximum dose of AraC chemotherapy, Nancy has been cruising through hospitalization two. Until today, she did not have any major side effects—though she has developed another blood clot and a skin infection. She is in the midst of her "bone marrow crash" due to the chemotherapy but remains positive and relatively strong.

Sincerely,

Winnie

An All-Too-Familiar Question

July 29, 7:20 p.m.

Dear Friends and Family,

There's a common question on the "penthouse" floor of LDS Hospital: *"How do you like my bald head?"*

No, the question wasn't from my Nancy. Our twenty-two-year-old friend Megan, the young woman fighting ovarian cancer, was readmitted to the hospital this morning and is once again our next-door neighbor. Megan's newest complication is a kidney infection, and she has returned to receive powerful IV antibiotics that must be monitored in the hospital. As a prelude to her first chemotherapy course, she has shaved her beautiful, very thick, very long, very dark hair. But the long strands will not go to waste. Megan has donated them to the American Cancer Society to have wigs made for young children with cancer.

After admission, our youthful friend laughed and didn't seem to mind when I walked over and rubbed her fuzzy round dome as I responded to her question, "I love it, Megan. In fact, I'm partial to bald-headed women. I know one in the next room who sends her best."

"How is Nancy?"

Even before I could answer, Megan closed her eyes, and in seconds, was asleep. The bed swallows her tiny frame; she was barely over one hundred pounds before her cancer and subsequent surgery—and now, she is probably just a little over eighty.

Several minutes later, Megan's eyes reopened. I knew to continue our conversation as if there had been no pause because

Nancy has done the same thing many times when chemotherapy or the disease (or both) have sapped her energy

"Nancy cruised through her second round of chemotherapy. It was much easier the second time around than it was the first."

My chest felt like my heart weighed a million pounds. (Megan's mother has told me the chemotherapy has started roughly.) I hope her experience in the second round will mirror Nancy's. Hopefully, Megan will go home tomorrow if there are no complications. Unlike Nancy, whose immune status precludes being outside the hospital, Megan is able to continue her treatment as an outpatient in the oncology clinic. Her prognosis remains very upsetting to me.

Summary: Please continue the positive energy for the next week or so as Nancy's immune status will be at its lowest. She and I both truly appreciate it. During the dark, lonely, or frightening times I try to focus on the love you send us. It makes all the difference in the world. Also, if you have anything left over, send it in Megan's direction.

With love,

Winnie

A Wait Well Worth It

August 6, 11:19 p.m.

Dear Friends and Family,

As a physician, it has been humbling to see how frequently patients "hurry up and wait." On an intellectual level, I was aware of the concept, but having been healthy, I had never experienced it up close and personal. I liken it to the difference between thinking about the experience of having a newborn baby versus sitting up all night in a rocking chair trying to get the little tyke to stop crying.

These last few months, I have learned firsthand about waiting. For example, when Nancy had a sore arm from her infection and blood clot during this hospitalization and was taking a strong pain medicine, it was, *"Winnie, has it been four hours yet since my last Percocet?"*

In reality, she didn't have to ask. The distressed expression on her beautiful face was already telling me it must be time for her next dose. The fact is that nothing is harder than watching a loved one suffer—except perhaps seeing that loved one and knowing what to do but being unable to "write the order."

It is considerably easier when Nancy asks, *"Do you see the lunch trays in the hall yet?"* My bride's voracious appetite this hospitalization is near legendary on the eighth floor. Nancy's desire for sustenance is much to the delight of her doctors and probably a result of her off-the-chart walking program.

Today, however, it was my turn to wait.

At 12:28 p.m. there was still no sign of our attending "main" doctor. I'd already missed breakfast and was beginning to worry that the hot lunch would be at room temperature by the time I reached the cafeteria. (Meals have become a welcome break to the monotony of watching the clock tick while Nancy sleeps.) Still I was afraid to leave; our chief physician was long overdue. For a moment my eyes closed, the memory of another fitful night on the hospital rollaway adding to the heaviness of my upper eyelids. Just as my stomach gurgled loud enough for it to be heard at the nurse's station down the hall, the door opened and in strolled Dr. Morton.

"I don't know how much of a hurry you are to get out of this prison room, Nancy, but I'm thinking maybe tomorrow. We'll decide in the morning when we see if your white count and platelets continue to go up. If they're just a little higher, we'll give you the boot. You'll have to take oral antibiotics for a day or so though."

Is Dr. Morton kidding?

Is it possible we'll be in our own comfortable bed by tomorrow evening?

"That okay with you two?" Dr. Morton raised his eyebrows while tilting his head forward.

Nancy's smile matched his. "That would be . . . GREAT."

Though most often not the case, this time my wait was well worth it.

Summary: With little notice, our doctor surprised us with an earlier than expected hospital discharge. Nancy is returning to our sanctuary by the river, where the flowers are still in full bloom and the birds are waiting to make the hospital noises a dim memory. Our upcoming two-week respite should be a fantastic escape. This time, Nancy is unencumbered by medical devices and, best of all, she feels great. Amazingly, she feels better now than when we entered the hospital nearly three weeks ago for round two.

Thanks for all your
love and support during
this last round,

Winnie

It's Party Time

August 10, 10:51 p.m.

Dear Friends and Family,

Nancy is in a really good place. She doesn't have any restrictions at this point, except to stay away from obviously ill people. Consequently, she wants to greet all of you who have helped so meaningfully with your kind words, thoughts, and deeds.

If you are free and can make it, we are having a small get-together on Sunday, August 14, between 1 p.m. and 4 p.m. at our home in Woodland.

Feel free to bring a fishing pole (if you like that sort of thing) because the Provo River runs alongside and through our property. (I'm told by those "in the know" that the rainbow trout are biting.)

Light refreshments will be provided, so please don't feel the need to bring anything.

We can't wait to see you!

Summary: Nancy shocked me this morning and had me send an invitation to our "local" supporters. Obviously, if any of you from greater distances want to witness my bride with a fuzzy head, you are more than welcome to drive or fly in. We have extra beds. And lots and lots of floor space.

Much love,

Winnie

The Numbers Don't Add Up, Part 1

August 12, 2:10 a.m.

Dear Friends and Family,

As promised in an earlier letter, I have some unpleasant news to relate. I've kept my medical update compartmentalized in a corner of my mind until I was feeling emotionally strong enough to bring it to the forefront.

Up until this point, I mostly live in the present. I concentrate on Nancy's upcoming meal, her current chemotherapy treatment, or an X-ray that may occur later in the day. Though I plan the next day each evening, I rarely address a future weekend or look ahead to when I might have two days off from work.

My "same-day-only" planning is about to change. Nancy and I are facing serious decisions. They are not straightforward or easy. There is a fork in the road regarding her care and we must choose which path to pursue.

Nancy has greatly enjoyed her home "vacation," especially since she feels "normal." Unlike the previous time she came home, she has not been tied to an IV or oxygen source. Being "unhooked" has allowed her to walk outside each day amid the trees and flowers, dine with her closest buddies at quiet restaurants, go shopping with Jayna, share popcorn with me at movies, and even host an open house attended by many of our local supporters. (For those of you who couldn't attend, the party was spectacular; Nancy beamed for hours and had a wonderful time seeing friends, both old and new.)

During the past week, while appearing to be carefree and fancy-free, we have been gathering information in order to decide whether to continue with three additional hospital-based chemotherapy courses or instead consider an unmatched (i.e., non-sibling) bone marrow transplant as soon as a donor can be identified.

To put our decision (and story) in context, we need to return to the day before Nancy left the hospital.

When he entered our room for his daily visit, Nancy greeted our Captain with, "Dr. Morton, I've been wanting to tell you something for a long time." Nancy paused, waiting until she was certain she commanded Dr. Morton's complete attention and he had pulled up a chair close to Nancy's bed: "You saved my life. Thank you."

"Captain" Morton, our oncologist, is tall, thin, and bespectacled. He appears more like a college professor than a doctor. (Of course, who am I to talk? I once was handed a broom while an intern in the hospital.) Though only in his early fifties, Dr. Morton has barely more hair than Nancy. He always speaks slowly and softly, thereby projecting a gentle demeanor. He'll discuss his golf game, his son in Portland, and Nancy's disease all in the same visit. True, Dr. Morton maintains an appropriate professional distance, but after two and a half months, there is a readily apparent fondness toward Nancy.

As a cancer specialist, Dr. Morton deals with suffering and death on an intimate and almost daily basis. He probably endures more patient deaths in a single month than I do in a decade. But when Nancy, in her straightforward and sincere manner, stated, "You saved my life. Thank you." Dr. Morton appeared to be in uncharted territory. His face turned bright red and he squirmed visibly in his chair.

"Uh . . . That's my job, Nancy. I'm sure your husband does the same kind of thing."

(I relate this conversation secondhand from Jayna, who called me at my day job in Park City when it occurred. Jayna sobbed as she related it.)

"Well, Winnie has saved a few people over the years," Nancy replied. "But not my life. If he was here, he'd thank you, too."

Dr. Morton started to speak but instead rose and made his way even closer to Nancy's bedside. Putting a hand on her shoulder, he smiled. Nancy returned his smile, a smile I can easily picture from Jayna's words: Glowing. Captivating. Intimate. And at that point, telling him it was all right to connect more than usual.

"Thank you, Nancy," he said in barely a whisper.

Nancy has always had a special influence on those around her.

I did arrive at the hospital in the early afternoon, in time to participate in a visit from Dr. Finn Bo Peterson, the transplant surgeon Dr. Morton had consulted, who quickly concluded, "After discussing your case with our team, we recommend you move to transplant as soon as possible."

Dr. Peterson explained that he had just reviewed Nancy's history, lab findings, and two hospital courses. But his conclusion was very different from what we had planned. In fact, it was totally different from what we expected. And most distressing, it was entirely different from what we had been told by Dr. Morton.

Dr. Morton's words from yesterday, when I was present for his visit, echoed in my mind: *"I recommend going through four courses of chemotherapy and saving any bone marrow transplant for what we call 'rescue therapy.' If you relapse, that's when to consider a transplant. I'm hoping you won't ever need one."*

The round of chemotherapy we are just now completing has gone relatively smoothly. Though Nancy did have a superficial blood clot and a secondary infection, we've been encouraged because she's feeling better and stronger than when she entered the hospital. She is poised to leave a full week ahead of schedule.

But now Dr. Peterson was presenting a wholly different opinion.

Hadn't Dr. Peterson talked with Dr. Morton?

Where I was speechless, Nancy wasn't: "Dr. Peterson, I'm confused. We've been operating under the assumption that a bone marrow transplant was saved for last. And only if things didn't work out. I think Dr. Morton called it 'rescue' therapy."

"Well, Nancy. If you have the four courses of AraC chemotherapy alone, unfortunately, you only have a 5–10% chance of survival."

Jayna and I looked at each other simultaneously, and a tear immediately rolled down her cheek.

What was this guy saying?

We'd just finally adjusted to and accepted the 30–40% chance Dr. Morton gave Nancy after we learned she was not in the 70% cure group for the M3 type of acute myeloid leukemia initially diagnosed.

How could the numbers change again?

How could they be so bad?

My face felt hot. My fingers tingled. Nancy was doing great, "cruising," according to Dr. Morton. He seemed excited when he anointed her his most "boring patient." In reality, I wanted to scream out loud. Instead, I gathered as calm a tone as I could muster and said, "Wait a minute, Dr. Peterson. I must be missing something? We've been told that Nancy has a 30–40% chance with just chemotherapy. Her leukemia seems very sensitive to the medicines." Although I consciously tried to suppress my emotions for Nancy, my voice did crack in the middle. Nancy nervously rubbed her arm.

Dr. Peterson was not fazed by my question or my cracking voice: "Well, Dr. Winn, sometimes there are different ways to look at data. With Nancy's age and the number of abnormal white cells in her blood when she first got sick, I believe that chemotherapy alone will not be successful."

After Dr. Peterson's response, I don't think I listened much.

Five to ten percent survival?

I vaguely recall Nancy confirming our insurance, acknowledging that her brother and sister's bone marrow tests hadn't matched, and discussing the next steps in moving toward a transplant. The process sounded long and tedious. I tried to concentrate but kept flashing on the 10% number. I just wanted to get to the end of this encounter.

When the meeting concluded and Dr. Peterson left, Jayna and Nancy didn't speak. Instinctively, the three of us hugged as a group, my left shoulder wet from Jayna's tears, my right from Nancy's.

Over two months into this ordeal, and it was only the third time I'd witnessed Nancy's tears.

I gently stroked Nancy's head, which was warm on my chest. She looked at me with still-moist eyes: "I'm so confused. I don't understand."

A single tear ran down her left cheek. "I was feeling positive."

How could things keep changing?

Why hadn't Dr. Morton and Dr. Peterson coordinated their stories?

How could we have been subjected to Dr. Peterson's interpretations without warning?

A simple "Dr. Peterson looks at things differently than I do. Don't be too alarmed if he uses different numbers and makes different recommendations. We'll discuss it later." would have been nice. Instead, just as we were cautiously proceeding down one path—we fell off a cliff.

No, we were pushed.

The three of us remained silent for what seemed an eternity. I paced the room trying to clear my head, to find a compartment for my anger and disappointment.

Should I call Dr. Morton right now or wait until his visit tomorrow?

I'm the "sleepover" person, I reasoned, and I don't work until 3:30 p.m. tomorrow at the clinic in Park City.

Can I make it until the morning feeling the way I do?

Remember, he saved her life, I told myself.

But how could this happen?

Nancy grabbed my arm as I passed by her bed: "Relax, Winnie. Sit beside me." Her eyes had regained their sparkle. And they were dry. Nancy laughed, "Look at you. I'm the one with the leukemia. We'll be fine."

Nancy poked me in the ribs until I begrudgingly laughed. Then she continued, "All right, I'm the leukie, not you. And I'm feeling pretty good, now that I think about it. Dr. Peterson said that with a transplant, my chance is 50–55%. Those are better odds than the 40% from Dr. Morton. He also said it didn't matter that Linda and Jim aren't able to donate marrow if we use the special procedure he plans. What did he call it?"

Before I could answer, Jayna did: "A mini-transplant, Mom." (Jayna watches Jeopardy every day with Nancy. I believe it's part of their closeness—part of their ritual. So she has lots of practice answering questions rapidly.)

I confirmed, "He did say that, Nancy. And it was a term I didn't recognize. I have lots of reading and research to do."

"Remember, Winnie, you're my husband—not the doctor."

"I know," I answered.

(I didn't add what I was also thinking—*more than you can imagine, my love.*)

Summary: This morning I shared part one of "how our lives are once again jumbled and twisted in every direction." I will compose part two early tomorrow.

Our best,

Winnie

The Numbers Don't Add Up, Part 2

August 13, 3:31 a.m.

Dear Friends and Family,

When Dr. Morton arrived the morning after our conversation with Dr. Peterson, his customary playful demeanor was absent. The lines around his eyes were tighter and there wasn't even a hint of a smile was on his lips.

"I understand Dr. Peterson from the transplant team came by yesterday. I've also heard he recommended a transplant right away."

News travels fast on the cancer floor.

Dr. Morton's statement is a testament to how deeply the oncology staff cares about all aspects of their patients' health. (The oncology floor functions like a big family.) After Dr. Peterson's visit, several on our team had noticed the dramatic, though transient, change in our family's attitude and disposition. And not only had they offered support, they apparently had related our concerns to our doctors.

Nancy smiled, something I was unable to do.

"He did. We were surprised."

"I'm sorry that happened, Nancy. I expected to talk to Dr. Peterson before he talked to you."

I chimed in, "It was distressing, Dr. Morton. His numbers were entirely different from the ones you gave us. His plan was entirely different as well. Nothing he said came close to what we had heard from you."

"Winnie, I'm sorry that I didn't talk to him first, and then you. I would have prepared you and Nancy had I known what he was thinking. Sometimes medicine is messy."

Messy?

That's for sure.

Still I had to respond: "Can you explain how you've advised us 30% to 40% for a survival estimate, yet he said 10–15%" (I refrained from adding, "To me, those numbers aren't even in the same galaxy.")

"We interpret the numbers differently. I can stand by mine, though I understand his conclusions"

What does that mean?

Doublespeak?

Oncology code? (Medical knowledge is often gray, but . . .)

"Dr. Morton, at this point, numbers don't mean much. They keep changing. We need advice. What should we do? Have you changed your mind on whether Nancy should get a transplant?"

"Well, Winnie, that's a fair question. I had a long discussion with Dr. Peterson on the subject this morning. He told me the newest studies don't support waiting, the way the old ones do. If Nancy has a relapse of her leukemia, it will be harder to get her back into remission while taking a heavy toll on her body. And she is fifty-seven years old. The chance of bone marrow success goes down as one approaches sixty. On the other hand, Nancy's leukemia has been very responsive. Plus, getting a transplant is tricky at best. It makes our chemotherapy treatments feel like a walk in the park."

How could a transplant be worse than our first hospitalization?

Remember, I told myself, he saved her life.

"Shouldn't we have been looking sooner for a match if we were even thinking about a transplant? Maybe we'd be ready now and not have to go through another chemotherapy course while we're waiting."

"I suppose we might have saved a week or two, Winnie. But it may take months to find an unmatched donor. In the big picture . . ."

In my small picture, every week counts. Every day counts!

Our meeting ended congenially enough, with Dr. Morton adding he forgot to mention that Nancy's pre-leukemic good health was a positive for the transplant side of the ledger and telling us that good health helped her with the chemotherapy, too.

He also had saved an encouraging note for the very last.

"I do have good news. You can go home tomorrow if Nancy's blood counts continue to rise."

Summary: Though the rebound of Nancy's blood counts will allow us to return to Woodland, a "homework" problem that may not have a clear answer has become part of our "vacation." Should we consider a transplant?

Love,

Winnie

It's as Clear as Mud

August 16, 11:11 p.m.

Dear Friends and Family,

A significant portion of our first week home has been spent negotiating the "insurance quagmire" as we consider if Nancy should attempt a bone marrow transplant, or BMT (also sometimes called a stem cell transplant). There are multiple forms for the many doctors to fill out, permissions and releases that are needed by the hospital and insurance company, and a never-ending myriad of phone calls. (The list is long, but I am persistent to say the least, and I can't help but wonder how someone with less understanding or determination can be expected to navigate such a detailed process.)

Even more important than the paperwork and financial aspects related to Nancy's hospitalization has been the identification of a suitable donor. (I believe I mentioned in an earlier note that Nancy, her brother Jim, and her sister Linda had their bone marrow "typed." Unfortunately, neither Linda nor Jim's bone marrow match Nancy's.)

Once I obtained the approval of the insurance company to proceed, the Human Lymphocyte Antigen (HLA) pattern (type) used to identify Nancy's unique bone marrow was sent to the National Marrow Donor Program. The process is sort of like a computer "dating" match for blood cells. After sending in the final paperwork yesterday, we only had to endure one restless night worrying. Today, we learned there were twenty-one potential donors. (Keep your fingers and toes crossed.)

Now the potential bone marrow donors will be contacted, questioned again about their present health and continued willingness, and then retested for the next set of more specific blood compatibility markers. This next phase can take from three weeks to six months. The process is a lot like Nancy's blood talking to the donor's blood and having several "dates" to see if a serious relationship is possible.

In the interim, if we decide to proceed with a transplant, the next question is where to do the procedure. In "transplant-speak," Nancy needs a MUD procedure. A MUD transplant is not dirty in any way; rather MUD is the abbreviation for matched unrelated donor. Only one local facility near Park City performs MUD transplants—the Huntsman Cancer Center, which is part of the University of Utah in Salt Lake City. Huntsman is a smaller transplant center than, for example, the Hutchinson Cancer Center in Seattle or the facility in Houston at MD Anderson Cancer Center.

So I have a new project.

What are the cure rates at these three locations?

What type (mini vs. full) of MUD transplants should we consider?

What are the "logistics" if we move Nancy and our family to Seattle or Houston?

Meanwhile, Nancy will undergo another round of chemotherapy to ensure she stays in remission while we figure all this out. And we will return to the "penthouse" floor of LDS Hospital in another six days. (I'd be struck by lightning if I told you I am ready.) In between all these tasks, our time at home has been filled with togetherness, fun, and peacefulness (when we are not thinking about the future).

Nancy has been exercising, eating, and mentally preparing for what lies ahead, while I have been constantly on the computer and phone. In all honesty, I am a wreck trying to sort through our next challenges, but Nancy has a different take: "I'm ready for the next round. After all, what's the alternative?" Somehow her sense of humor will drag me back to the rollaway on the eighth floor, smiling and willingly.

Lastly, I would be remiss by not mentioning that we are fortunate to have some physician cousins on my side of the family. (Thank you, Sam and Richard.) Invaluably, they are helping me contact out-of-state experts for their opinions on which procedure might be best and where to obtain treatment. I suspect the decision will not be clear cut and will require a certain amount of "best guessing" on what feels right.

Which is where all of you come in.

Your constant support and energy continues to give us the resolve to forge forward and the strength to choose a direction.

Summary: It has been great to be home with Nancy feeling so good. Especially since it has been time to decide if we should proceed with a transplant, what kind of transplant we should choose, and where we should have it.

Thanks and love,

Winnie

The Details Are a Little Muddy

August 18, 11:01 p.m.

Dear Friends and Family,

After my most recent letter, many of you have inquired about becoming a bone marrow (stem cell) donor. So this letter is specifically for you, though Nancy and I have no expectations of our friends. For everyone else, feel free to skip the details.

Here is what I have surmised from the growing pile of materials we've received.

Be The Match®, operated by the National Marrow Donor Program, is the largest and most diverse bone marrow registry in the world. It is a nonprofit organization dedicated to helping every patient get the life-saving transplant they need.

Joining the Be The Match Registry is easy. Just log on to their website at BeTheMatch.org, where you will find all the pertinent information about becoming a registered potential donor. You can even click "Join" to join the registry immediately by providing your birthdate and general medical information. When they ask for a promotion code, if you type in "Nancy" we will be notified that you have become a donor. A kit will be mailed to you that contains a couple of swabs to obtain cells from the inside of your cheeks to send back to the registry. From those cells, the donor's specific immunogenic profile, called HLA typing, becomes part of a national database that can be accessed for patients needing a transplant. Donors between eighteen and forty-four are preferred and no financial contribution is required. Donors between forty-five and sixty can join, but a financial contribution of $100 is requested to offset the cost of the testing.

There are currently over twenty-five million people already registered in the program, and a Caucasian has a high likelihood of finding a match from the current bank of traditional HLA immunologic screening samples.

When a donor's blood is tested and found to have the same HLA fingerprints, it is called a match.

When a transplant doctor requests typing for his patient, it usually takes only one day to check the central computer for potential matches, and when they are found, the names are then sent back to the requesting doctor and transplant center.

The doctor next asks the registry to contact the potential donors to see if they are still available and willing and to do further, more specific testing.

New antigens are discovered each year, and further testing refines an unmatched donor's sample to see if it is even more closely similar to the recipient's.

Additionally, a donor is screened for infectious diseases that could prevent a successful transplant—for example, HIV, cytomegalovirus, or one of the hepatitis viruses.

What is the chance you would be a match with Nancy?

It is rare that a non-sibling donor match has been discovered by having a friend's cells tested. One of those times was in a tribal setting from a close ethnic group and therefore a higher probability.

So in reality, it is highly unlikely.

It is a testimony to your kindness and caring to realize that (any of) you have considered this process. And we are most appreciative.

If you follow this procedure, you might help someone like Nancy in the future. Also, more immediate help for Nancy and others with similar problems will occur with a blood or platelet donation that can be done in Nancy's name. Patients like Nancy require multiple platelet and blood transfusion during the periods they are receiving strong chemotherapy.

But again, we have no expectations.

And we thank you from the bottom of our hearts just for asking.

Summary: Since so many of you have inquired about how to be a bone marrow donor, I've summarized how you might be able to help Nancy or someone like her.

With much love,

Winnie

The Large and Small of It All

August 19, 4:50 a.m.

Dear Friends and Family,

As promised, a few more words about the party we hosted last week.

When Nancy graduated from the University of Georgia with a teaching degree, she decided to take a year off to become a flight attendant and see "the world outside of Georgia." She chose the international carrier Trans World Airlines (TWA) instead of interviewing with Atlanta-based Delta like many of her friends. Not surprisingly, TWA recognized a "quality" individual and immediately hired Nancy, thereby beginning a thirty-three-year career of travel and adventure while based in various cities such as New York, Boston, St. Louis, and Los Angeles. She definitely wasn't in Georgia anymore (or Kansas for that matter).

During her first extended independent living experience, Nancy secured an apartment in the town of Long Beach on New York City's Long Island, an easy drive to Kennedy Airport, where most of her flights originated. It wasn't long before she and her roommate, Julie, made friends and decided to host a dinner party for two male coworkers. Decades later Julie told me an important detail about that night: "Winnie, it was probably the most embarrassing night of my life. Even though we cooked most of the day, we didn't have enough food." (Those few sentences still elicit hysterical and prolonged laughter from Julie and Nancy whenever they reminisce.)

On a tight budget, they apparently didn't realize how much young men (or "boys" as they were deemed) can eat. Both

Nancy and Julie kept retreating to the kitchen to find some-thing, anything to add to their dates' plates, which the boys all but licked clean. Nancy told me many years later that neither girl actually ate a bite so they could secretly switch their food to the boys' plates.

I believe that one dinner party has easily doubled our fami-ly's grocery bills over the years whenever we entertain. It is not uncommon to have a week's worth of leftovers every time we have company, even after Nancy sends any remaining desert home with our guests.

You can only imagine, then, what our house looked like when Nancy invited people to visit us during her recent home "vacation." Every small shelf or corner overflowed with chips, nuts, candy, cheese, crackers, and other snacks. Every coffee and end table accommodated brightly colored fresh flowers. Our dining room table and kitchen counters had countless entrees of fish, meat, potatoes, salads, and vegetables. Our bar was the main drink area, and not one person asked for a drink that I couldn't provide in a moment's notice. I know that we had leftovers for all our remaining days home and then some.

Still I had no regrets.

Each step of the planning, cleaning, shopping, setting up, and cooking was enjoyable. This was Nancy's first face-to-face contact with most of her "local" friends. This was Nancy's first contact with a "feeling" community.

The most ordinary tasks seemed almost special. Nancy's declaration, while vacuuming the living room, echoed how Jayna, Jaret, and I felt as we whipped our house into "party" readiness. She declared, "I never thought I'd say this, but vac-uuming can be fun." (On her last visit home, Nancy had been too weak for such a task.)

The night before the party, after trying on most everything in her closet to select the "best" outfit, Nancy and Jayna took up most of our bed while they talked over final plans. "It's like the night before the prom, Dadder. Mom is nervous." Jayna kissed her mother's head as we all twittered like children, alone together sharing intimate thoughts.

When 2 p.m. arrived the next day and her guests arrived at our doorstep, Nancy was glowing. Except for the brightly colored scarf that Jayna fashioned over Nancy's now fuzzy head, it was difficult to tell that Nancy was just on a "time out" from her deathly illness. Everyone treated her normally, and for three hours she looked and felt that way. The only tears that were shed were by me, when I sneaked away to our bedroom, overcome by watching Nancy be so happy and so alive.

It was a momentous day—both large and small.

Nancy, in talking to my partner Joe Ferriter's eight-months-pregnant wife, Jenny, inquired about what they were planning for childcare since Jenny was also a physician. Upon finding some uncertainty, she paired Jenny with our dear friend Mona, a retired preschool teacher who was looking for something to do part time.

Problem solved.

Typical Nancy.

Summary: The highlight of our time home has been the chance for Nancy to visit with friends while feeling good. It was a truly extraordinary gathering.

All my love,

Winnie

That's a Lot of Stuff

September 1, 11:07 p.m.

Dear Friends and Family,

I find it hard to believe it has been almost two weeks since I last wrote you. Either I am getting used to the roller coaster ride or I have been overwhelmed by the responsibilities of my day job in Park City—plus my attempt to keep our family on an even keel.

It is not easy to live in a hospital room, watching Nancy endure her next round of chemotherapy.

Am I numb or exhausted? Or both?

Many days I don't know. Anyway, Nancy is laboring along, already one week into this "visit" to our hospital home.

So how did this round begin?

"Now that's a lot of stuff," I heard from a voice to my left.

I turned to view the round face of a plump, fortyish woman. Her head was tilted in my direction to get a maximum look at the many items in the extra-large blue storage bin riding on the arms of the wheelchair that I had borrowed from the check-in desk at the hospital. Six clumps of plastic flowers were proudly sticking their yellow, red, and blue tops from the second of our two bins that was being transported to Nancy's new eighth-floor room. Numerous books, pictures, clothing, stuffed animals, and other various sentimental items were directly visible to this all-too-curious lady's view. (I bought the bins at Staples at the end of our first hospitalization, and the containers have allowed us to move in and out of the hospital with ease and efficiency, albeit not with much privacy.)

"My wife will be here a long time. Probably a month," I responded, trying to talk to her and not to the other folks in

152

the elevator who now were looking at the bin directly rather than glancing at it fleetingly so as not to stare.

"Oh . . . ," the lady replied, shuffling her feet nervously. "I'm very sorry." The lady literally ran off the elevator when we reached the fourth floor, not meeting my eyes or even saying good-bye. The fourth floor is the newborn floor; she was probably a new grandmother, I concluded. The patient she would visit probably would stay in the hospital two days at the maximum.

Feeling somewhat self-conscious, I looked at the ceiling mirror as I transported "a lot of stuff" the final four floors to the "penthouse." The other visitors on the elevator marched off at intermediate floors, looking at their feet just like the "curious" lady. By the seventh floor, I was finally alone.

Why do I feel uncomfortable on a hospital elevator?

A month is a long time to be quarantined in a room that is drab and antiseptic by design. Jayna and I have made every effort to fill Nancy's room with fun things, to add a personal touch to offset and soften the absence of personal decor. We want Nancy to be surrounded in all directions with reminders from friends and family. One card hanging on a wall might bring to mind ten emails or letters I've read to her.

(Each of you has touched Nancy's heart in countless ways; I want your love nearby during the hard times.)

Once off the elevator, I spent the next hour framing the already existing pictures with our bendable plastic flowers, filling the bulletin board with thumb-tacked mementos and cards, and placing Nancy's growing "herd" of stuffed animals in every corner and on every shelf.

Nancy assumes the director role on "move-in" day and isn't hesitant to point out, "No, I like it better over there. Like last time." Though Nancy feigns objection at so much fuss, I suspect deep down inside she likes her room's renovation.

By the time I empty both bins, the all-white room had been transformed into a menagerie of color. Our plastic flowers offer no smell, but Nancy speculates proudly that our room has as much foliage as exists in the entire hospital. And certainly, it has the most cards and pictures. As a last gesture, Jayna opens a perfume bottle and dabs it all around the room to block out the smell of bleach and soap. I like the fragrant smell almost as much as its name: *Eternity*.

Each and every one of the staff on our first day back made a comment: "You've transformed this room into a garden paradise again. And look at these new pictures. Are they from your party?" Jane, one of Nancy's nurses during her past two hospitalizations, turned to Jayna and shared an observation that touched us greatly: "Everyone on our staff loves coming to your room. You make it home."

For the first time in a while, I can remember that things do matter. Earlier I was frantic when I thought I had misplaced the beagle stuffed animal given to Jaret by his great Uncle Hank. "Hushpuppy" is one of Nancy's favorites. She expects him to be sitting on our tiny windowsill in Room 842, like always.

Funny what really matters on day one of hospitalizations.

Summary: We're back on the penthouse floor. Room 842. And we brought a lot of stuff with us to make it our home—for now.

> With love from Hushpuppy, our many other stuffed companions, and Nancy,
>
> Winnie

New Stories from Cancerland

September 9, 3:42 a.m.

Dear Friends and Family,

A story from yesterday.

"All right Winnie, visualization time." Our nurse for the day, Wendy, has just hung Nancy's chemotherapy medicine. Nancy closes her eyes, but I'm not ready and I can only look at her. Some place deep inside her body, she is fighting a battle.

Is it the "Pac-Men" eating the "bad" guys?

Soldiers in white against soldiers in red or black?

A gold potion or a magical wand?

Nancy is in her zone, imagining her Vitamin C (our nickname for the AraC, chemotherapy drug) searching out any residual leukemia cells. But on the outside, there is no battle. Nancy looks beautiful. Relaxed. Peaceful. My bride's fuzzy dome sparkles in the early morning sunlight that streams through our tiny mountain-facing window. I want to rub that head, just like I do so many times each day.

Before I decide if such a foolish action might break her concentration, there is a telltale sound. A snort. This now all-too-familiar noise is the prelude to Nancy snoring, which occurs seconds later. Her battle is over. I'm certain she's won; she's now fast asleep.

The medicine continues to run, barely halfway finished. The powerful chemotherapy drug, still flowing into the new central IV line just below Nancy's right clavicle, needs my help. I close my eyes. I pick up the baton from Nancy. It is my turn for adventures (and battles) in Cancerland.

I think I'll imagine gladiators this time.

One story from today.

Schedules. Though I attempt to live in the present, I sometimes am forced to plan a few days in advance. For example, I
knew that last Tuesday and Wednesday, I wasn't going to have
to work in Park City. Therefore, for those entire two days and
nights, Nancy would find me by her side or just south of her feet.

Thursday, however, was a different story. My day job at the
clinic would require my attendance. I was scheduled for the
late 12:30–9:00 p.m. shift as well as being on call. By the time
I realized my problem, it was too late to trade shifts. Jayna,
unfortunately, was asleep at Woodland after having spent more
than twenty-four hours traveling back from Peru, where she
had attended the wedding of her boyfriend's brother. Though
her travel was free (as a result of Nancy's past employment),
several of the planes from Dallas to Salt Lake City had been
full, and Jayna had spent the previous night stretched out on
an airport bench, attempting to sleep. For that reason, she was
"out for the count" Tuesday and Wednesday. Thursday wasn't
any better either. It was her first day of school at the University of Utah, and she would have to be gone at least part of the
day—if not all of it. To make matters even worse, Linda was
back in Georgia teaching ESL.

After only a brief pause, I somewhat hesitantly picked up the
phone: "Jaret, what would you think of spending the day with
Mom on Thursday? You'll just have to be with her until Jayna
finishes school and gets her books."

Jaret had stayed alone with his mom once before without a
problem. Still I was hesitant about putting him in a position
where he might be uncomfortable. He still hated blood. He
didn't like me to talk about diseases with Jayna. In reality, he
pretty much avoided everything medical—especially hospitals.
Growing up, I all-too-well remember him saying, "Hospitals
give me the creeps, Dad. I don't know how you do it."

Without a second's hesitation, Jaret answered, "Dad, it's my
turn. And I can sleep over, too. I want to help Mom. And you."

And so it was that Jaret had his first "sleepover" with Nancy.

When I finally made it home around midnight and climbed
between the sheets exhausted, I tossed and turned. I worried
about Jaret not sleeping. I worried if his presence was a strain

for Nancy, who needs every bit of sleep she can get. Instead, Jaret answered Nancy's phone when I nervously called the next morning for a progress report.

"It wasn't a big a deal, Dad. I slept really well. And Mom did, too. Didn't you, Mom?" Pride radiated from my son like the mouthwatering smell emanating from a kitchen on Thanksgiving. And I truly and thankfully appreciated it just as much.

Summary: Jaret continues to grow and mature. Not everything about Nancy having leukemia has been bad. Some things have been good.

Much love,

Winnie

Smiles All Around

September 9, 11:05 p.m.

Dear Friends and Family,

During my silent period, I forgot to relate a most important fact.

So another story from our first day back in the hospital.

Each day, Dr. Morton makes his rounds during one of two time periods. Round one begins at 9 a.m. before his office hours. And round two, around 5:30 p.m. after his office workday ends. Consequently, this morning when the clock read twenty after nine, it was looking like I wouldn't see him until the end of the day. (I didn't mean to be impatient, but Nancy's bone marrow report was most likely sitting atop his office desk.)

On the day of our return for hospitalization three, Nancy had once again quietly endured the big, long needle being thrust deeply into her right hip. The grinding sound, though familiar, was no less chilling even though Nancy didn't wince or squeeze my hand any harder than the last time. But the wait seemed harder this time around, and we both wanted to know the results.

Is she still in remission?

Would Dr. Morton at least call if it were bad news?

Shouldn't he want to call if it was good news?

I found myself repeatedly looking at the clock. When the big hand was on the four and the little one nearest the nine, I made my decision. I wouldn't wait until after his workday. I wanted to know now.

I decided to sneak out into the hall so that Nancy wouldn't know I was worried. And if the results weren't favorable, then I could figure out how to deliver disappointing news. My concern was caused by the fact that the day before the test, Nancy had seemed tired. And two days before that she bled slightly while flossing her teeth. (My teeth bleed too, but I don't have leukemia.) But before I could put my plan into action, there was a familiar knock on our door at twenty-two minutes after nine.

"Hi, Nancy, how is my most boring patient today."

Nancy awakened quickly. "I'm fine, Dr. Morton. How are you?" Nancy and the "Captain" connected with big, warm grins.

I didn't smile. I wanted the news first.

"Well, first off I want to tell you about your bone marrow. There was no leukemia. That's exactly what I hoped for—and expected. But it's always nice to get that report. What do you think of that, Winnie?"

I didn't speak. I was certain he could read my beaming face.

I'm still smiling. After two weeks in the hospital, our second home, things are so far, so good.

Summary: We are amid hospitalization three and have fantastic news. The bone marrow test Nancy endured for this round confirms that she is still in remission.

Thanks for your
thoughts and prayers
and for continuing to
remember us,

Winnie

The Perfect Vacation

September 12, 10:48 p.m.

Dear Friends and Family,

Numerous times during this journey I have used the word "vacation."

To date, "vacation" has meant the time Nancy and I spend in between her treatments and hospitalizations at our beloved home in the mountains. "Vacation" has seemed an apt term, as any time away from toxic medicines that make Nancy sick and threaten her life is certainly an escape, retreat, or holiday in the world of leukemia.

On the other hand, the last seven days have been a "traditional" vacation for me because I was "off" from my day job in Park City. Today is the last day of that vacation. Even so, I awoke feeling warm and fuzzy.

What was the first thing I saw this morning?

In the bed beside my rollaway, I mostly observed an overstuffed royal-blue quilt, the treasured present from Nancy's dear college friend from Minnesota, Patricia McCleese. As happens with Nancy and quilts, the comforter engulfed Nancy's body. The only part of Nancy I can monitor is a sweet little head surrounded by a halo of pillows. She is still asleep, looking thoroughly serene. I tiptoe closer to capture the moment. Nancy's hair is once again growing, some of it is over an inch in length and no longer sticking straight up. I still can't discern the dominant color, but it makes me chuckle to myself all the same just to see the stubble burst forth in every possible direction like Nancy had placed her finger in an electric socket.

"What?" Nancy says with a start. I gaze into her sleepy eyes but get lost in their sky-blue radiance. I find myself wondering, did Patricia know how well the quilt would highlight her eyes?

"Good morning, darlin'," I say, as has become my best "southern" custom.

Nancy yawns, then shuts her eyes. She is back in dreamland.

Will she remember?

The tired ache deep in my bones has disappeared because my only duties have been those having to do with the hospital. I have not worked for nearly a week. I have not had to race between the clinic in Park City and the hospital in Salt Lake City, changing roles and sometimes clothes in the Subaru. I feel both rested and invigorated.

Watching Nancy breathe normally, I am thankful. She displays no effort. In this same room during her first hospitalization, she struggled to breathe. The image is hard to erase. But so are the tricks that, at times, several of Nancy's drugs play with her mind.

A vacation in the hospital "penthouse"?

Where else but the "penthouse" is every meal brought to your room?

Where else is the service completely personalized?

Everyone in this hospital knows you and you are treated as if you are staying in a fine hotel. Everyone really and truly cares about you and your family. On a daily basis, you have long conversations with staff. You get to know about them, too. Jane has three kids, with one young adult in college. Will likes to mountain bike.

Do I ask too many questions?

Time has seemed suspended this week—almost nonexistent. Not once were Nancy and I in a rush. We took leisurely walks twice a day, we talked on the phone to friends and family, we read your emails, notes, letters, and parts of books, and we watched videos and the ever-present TV game shows. The days were wonderfully lazy. I was always there during Nancy's best times of the day. I was always there during her worst times of the day, too.

Nancy, with me by her side to monitor how she looked and felt, decided this week that it was all right for friends to stop by for a brief hello. There was more merriment in our room than in all the weeks that have recently passed. (Friends never visited us in Hawaii or Europe or South America during our other vacations.)

There was no dealing with airports or taxis or crowds. (How wonderful is that?) A vacation without travel hassles. (And how could I forget?) It's fall now. Our view of the mountains is spectacular. Even through our tiny little window.

In all honesty, I did miss having a beach, or at least a pool and hot tub. And we didn't get to walk through a jungle or browse a museum. Our strolls were limited to a circle around the eighth floor of the hospital; Nancy strode the halls decked out in her robe and her pink Boston Red Sox cap, wearing a protective mask. (Quite the fashion icon. Thanks, John. She loves the good luck hat.) And we all-too-well now know every picture, sign, and crack in the wall along our well-traveled path.

True, our "penthouse" room at LDS Hospital is not as nice as the least expensive room at a Marriott. But in our "home," we are able to do our own decorating. We are completely surrounded by things of our choosing. In my mind, the decor beats the Bellagio hands down.

Nancy has room service for every meal, while my food comes mostly from the twenty-four-hour cafeteria. It is not gourmet, but it is both cheap and plentiful. Nancy's room and board is more expensive than any first-rate room in the world. But I stay free, even though I am not a child. And it's likely insurance will pay for most of this "vacation." That's never happened before at a Hilton.

A different vacation for me?

Yes. Though I sometimes feel sad, lost, and even despondent. I have done more thinking about life's mysteries than on any previous ten vacations. Plus, when I add everything up, I have had quality time (and lots of it) with the love of my life.

And by the way, if you don't know it by now, Nancy could turn a jail cell into a holiday.

Summary: I had a week's vacation from my "day job" and spent it entirely in the "penthouse" with Nancy. She feels good. Our vacation was perfect.

Best,

Winnie

Two Is Better than One

September 13, 5:06 a.m.

Dear Friends and Family,

Dr. Peterson paid an unexpected visit to our LDS Hospital "home" last week while Nancy was in the midst of her latest round of chemotherapy: "I've talked to six respected oncologists around the country, none of them transplant surgeons. They're evenly split 50/50 on which way to go."

(I am sure that I don't have to remind you that our first visit with Dr. Peterson had been a disaster. After he informed us that Nancy's chance of survival without a bone marrow transplant was 10–15%, it had been all but impossible for me to listen to another word. I had been too stunned to ask a single question. Now after researching transplants and talking to lots of outside sources, I was prepared.)

"Then you have a different view of our situation from when we talked last?"

I'd waited nearly five weeks to hear his answer.

"Yes, Dr. Winn, I do. I've had a chance to study Nancy's case in greater depth, and I have consulted with others in the field. Quite simply, there's no clear-cut recommendation for you and your wife. When we talked before, I gave you a number based on Nancy's age and disease. But as you know, Nancy's been atypical. Her response to initial chemotherapy has been more rapid and better than expected, so her chances are probably better than I previously thought. Unfortunately, there aren't enough cases like hers to give you more exact statistics."

Though not a specific number, I was pleased to hear that his perception of Nancy's chances was better than the last time we talked. Nancy and I weren't shy with our questions.

"What is the cure rate at your facility for someone Nancy's age?"

"Which drugs do you use?"

"Will she require radiation?"

"What qualifications does someone need to work on your floor?"

"Can family members stay the whole time?"

The queries we posed Dr. Peterson went on and on. We inquired about staffing levels, projected time frames, and our most pressing question—which type of transplant Nancy might have if we proceeded with surgery.

"Do you recommend a full or mini-transplant?"

Dr. Peterson answered each question patiently and was not afraid to say, as he often did, "I don't know." He came across as both caring and thoughtful. He appeared both knowledgeable and competent. He good-naturedly answered questions for more than an hour. I was excited and satisfied about gaining so much knowledge. After shaking Dr. Peterson's hand and thanking him for coming, I turned to Nancy. It was only then that I noticed wrinkles of distress stretched across her brow.

"What's the matter, Nancy?"

"Oh, nothing much. Really." (Southern speak, even to me.)

"That's not what your face says."

Nancy reached out her hand for me to hold. "I thought I knew what I needed to do, Winnie. I was prepared for a transplant, even though it sounds horrible. Now I don't know."

How could I have been so stupid?

Nancy needed a narrow focus, a clear direction. I'd asked too many questions, and many of Dr. Peterson's answers, though honest, highlighted that we were in uncharted waters. We were in an unknown sea with waves crashing all around us. I had made a big and unforgivable mistake. I'd allowed Nancy to see the uncertainty of her treatment.

"I am so sorry, Nancy." I wanted to cry, scream, to somehow rewind the meeting. I wanted to start the meeting over, in the hall—without Nancy. I'd decided on my own that a transplant was a viable option and that Salt Lake City had a respectable program with a good leader. I knew inherently that Nancy, like me, was impressed with Dr. Peterson.

I simply didn't know what to say.

"Nancy, think of it this way. We have two good options, not just one. If they don't find a match for you, we still have a reasonable chance . . ."

I'd run out of words. I'd messed up. Nancy now looked more concerned—not less. I hugged her upper body that was limp in my arms. Minutes passed.

"Winnie, it's time for you to go. Jayna will be here any minute and I don't want you to be late for your ride."

Already, Nancy had shifted gears. She was worried that I might miss my daily mountain bike ride with Chuck English in Park City.

"But . . ."

"No buts. Get going. I need some alone time."

So did I.

My mobile phone rang just as I was leaving the Salt Lake City valley, starting the climb toward Parley's Summit. I couldn't help but notice that the mountain pass was already covered by scrub oak displaying multiple shades of red—a harbinger of fall. A familiar caller ID appeared as I answered, "Hey, sweetheart. What's happening? Are you all right? Do you forgive me?"

"Winnie, I love you more than I can say. And I want you to know that I'm fine. I've recovered. We have two good options. I accept that. I'm sure one of our two options will make itself clear to us. And I'll be ready."

Thirty minutes later, I arrived in Park City. My spirits had risen more quickly than the mountain road that connected my hospital "home" with my real "home." The newly colored leaves were even more vibrant at the higher elevation and their beauty mesmerized me. My phone rang again. The same caller ID appeared on the screen.

"Guess what I just did, Winnie? I rode the exercise bike for half an hour."

Nancy's report magnified her previous words. She was communicating in a different way—*I'll be ready.* Once again, worrying about me. Once again, giving reassurance.

Nancy is more beautiful than the leaves of fall.

Summary: We talked with the transplant surgeon. We really liked him and what he had to say. Our decision is not yet clear-cut. Neither of our two options—continue chemotherapy or undergo a bone marrow transplant—is, in Nancy's case, clearly better. Thanks for your ongoing and continued encouragement. It will give us the needed strength to move forward together.

Love,

Winnie

In Search of Mecca

September 28, 11:35 p.m.

Dear Friends and Family,

My apologies.

It has been awhile since I've written you, but this update is positive.

Nancy made it through her six doses of AraC with no untoward effects. Similar to last time, her AraC chemotherapy caused a bone marrow crash, leaving her immunocompromised and anemic. (Just as it is supposed to do.)

Tomorrow Nancy will return home and there is other good news, too.

Nancy feels relatively decent. Even though this was her third round of "poisons" (as chemotherapy drugs are nicknamed), her stay this time was uneventful and benign. As before, there will be no oxygen tubes or IV medicines during our home "vacation." Her medical team does plan to leave a permanent IV line entering Nancy's right upper chest. (Thankfully, for now, it's inactive.) The only reminder that she's survived another bout with her life-threatening disease will be the changing of her IV dressing once a day. (That, of course, and the cute, fuzzy head Nancy will see when she looks in the mirror.)

The other evening as our entire family was celebrating the final night of round three, Jayna put it very simply: "Mom rocks. She's got this chemo thing down."

What's next?

Our transplant pursuit continues as we await news of a willing and more refined match from the twenty-one potential donors identified by the National Marrow Donor Program.

When (and if) we receive word that Nancy has a bone marrow match from an unknown donor, we will have three questions to address:

1. Do we attempt the transplant or instead do two more rounds of chemotherapy?

2. If we decide to go for a BMT (bone marrow transplant), do we undergo what is termed a "full" transplant versus a less toxic procedure called a "mini-transplant"?

3. If we do go the transplant route, where (the University of Utah in Salt Lake City vs. far away from home) do we go?

Each question is serious. Each question has major implications.

As we get ready to leave for home tomorrow, Nancy is feeling about as normal as anyone can with leukemia. Before this last hospitalization, another negative bone marrow test confirmed that Nancy is still in remission. Being in remission is essential to any decision. And being in remission means there is still a chance to overcome whatever long or longer odds we face.

At this point, if we could write our own script, we'd continue indefinitely along our current path. We'd spend three quarter of our days on the Cancerland floor of the hospital doing treatments and spend the balance of our days in Woodland. (We would still call it "vacation.")

Even though our lives would have changed drastically, we'd never look back. We could be satisfied with our current routine and not ask for anything more.

As long as Nancy is not suffering . . .

However, we don't have that choice.

It's time to look forward.

It's time to think and plan.

It's time to not only consider but also choose.

We will do our utmost to determine which treatment best fits Nancy and our family. A big decision is no longer an undertaking for the future.

The time is now.

On October 2, Nancy and I will seek a second opinion at the world's largest transplant center, the Fred Hutchinson Cancer Center in Seattle, Washington. It's a bit frightening to know that Nancy will have to transit through two airports filled with lots of people and their accompanying germs.

Our trip will be uncomfortable for Nancy. Her hair is still nonexistent. She will be self-conscious about an IV line that could be visible unless she wears clothing that hides it. There will be many issues and problems that I can't yet imagine.

My first cousin Dr. Richard Winn, the chairman of neuro-surgery at the University of Washington, has arranged for us to meet with his friend Dr. Fred Appelbaum, a world-renowned bone marrow transplant expert and deputy director at the Cancer Center—the birthplace of bone marrow transplants. The center is widely regarded as the "Mecca" for blood cancer research and treatment. We are hoping that Dr. Appelbaum will have answers to our questions.

Both our attending oncologist (Dr. Morton) and our local transplant specialist (Dr. Peterson) have polled other experts regarding the two treatment options: continuing with chemo-therapy only or, if a good match can be found, undergoing a transplant. Unfortunately, the respondents were divided about equally. This leaves us with even more questions than when we began our journey.

Will Dr. Appelbaum tip the balance?

Will he be able to answer which type of transplant is best for Nancy?

Will we need to relocate our family to Seattle?

Tough questions will be a fundamental part of our difficult trip ahead. However, in the intervening time, we'll savor the splendor of fall in the Uinta Mountains, hoping these next two weeks are filled with bright sunshine, colored leaves, and our dearest of friends.

Summary: Though it is risky, Nancy and I will travel to Seattle in a few days to meet with the transplant experts at the world's original and most famous transplant center.

With love,

Winnie

Perfection Is in the Numbers

September 29, 8:13 p.m.

Dear Friends and Family,

Today is Nancy's first full day home.

As is my usual habit, I woke up this morning at 7 a.m. My face was warmed by bright sunshine streaming through the sliding glass doors that make up the south side of our bedroom, as I lay in bed quietly not wanting to wake Nancy and thinking about where life has taken me in the past months of Nancy's illness. I felt rested, more so than in weeks. Together, Nancy and I were in our bed. We were comfortable together. There had been no interruptions for vital signs. There had been no pills or blood work to awaken us at 5 a.m. There had been no sounds outside our room, save the sweet gurgling of the brook just beyond the deck. I wasn't surprised that Nancy was still asleep.

After a while, I decided to embrace the luxury of laziness, so I simply watched Nancy dream for the better part of a half hour. It is a beautiful sight to see her peacefully breathe in a normal fashion. I daydreamed about the many things she and I might do today. Thinking about the simple rhythms of our life together and the freedom of being home almost brought me to tears.

When the sunlight crept to her side of the bed, Nancy opened her eyes. I rubbed her head. "Good morning, sweetheart. What are your thoughts on the day?"

"I want to feel what it's like to walk places without dragging an IV pole around. I want to go there." Nancy pointed toward the glass doors through which we could see the flowers on the deck and the grove of aspens at the river's edge.

"But I do have one thing to do today. I have to go to Salt Lake City and help Jaret with a paper that's due tomorrow. It's funny, I'm really looking forward to the drive down to the city. It will be exhilarating to drive again."

"Okeydokey. Then turn away from the sun and take another nap. I'm going to make you breakfast and serve it to you in bed."

"What are your plans, Winnie?"

My mind replied, "To whisk you off to Morocco for a ride on a camel."

Unfortunately, my mouth conveyed a completely different comeback: "I have a dentist appointment this afternoon, and after that I'm planning to ride with Chuck. I might get my hair trimmed if Stephanie can fit me in. I need to stop at the bank . . ."

So much for being lazy, I mused, "Oh . . . And if you can believe it, Emmy is making us dinner again, so I'll pick that up while I'm in Park City. I could also make a DVD run if you are up for it. How does that sound?"

"Great. All of it."

Mundane, day-to-day stuff. It's hard to believe. Things seem so normal.

Not long ago, we started a new early morning tradition that I've hinted at in previous notes. I now give Nancy countless small kisses across her fuzzy dome each day. "These are sent from your friends," I tell her, though truth be known, at least half are from me. I give her only one hug, though I make it a very long one to reflect the many friends who end their conversations with me not by saying "Good-bye"—but instead declaring, "Give Nancy a hug for me."

This morning, as I wrapped Nancy in my arms, I noticed her eyes close and her mouth form a large grin. And just as I unwrapped my arms and gave Nancy a final kiss, the phone rang.

"Good morning, Winnie. This is Rachael Beers from the Transplant Unit at the University of Utah. I hope I'm not calling too early."

Too early? (Even a 5 a.m. call would be welcomed from Rachael. I have faithfully been contacting her each day the last few weeks, hoping for any news about a possible donor.)

"I believe that in our last conversation I told you that of the twenty-one potential matches for Nancy identified by the

National Marrow Donor Program, I requested seven for the next round of tests. Only five were still available and three didn't make the next cut—but two did. The last time we talked, those samples were undergoing the final analysis."

My heart was pounding as Rachael paused.

"I've got good news, Winnie. We have our donor."

What does it feel like to win the lottery? A number of years ago, I watched a TV show about winners, but in all honesty, I was simply not able to grasp the concept. Now I fully and completely understand.

As Rachael uttered, "We have our donor," my pulse accelerated and total exhilaration took over. My body trembled and goose bumps appeared everywhere. I effusively and totally embraced Nancy. My hug this time was only from me.

Rachael continued, "I am allowed to tell you the donor is a male. More importantly, he's a 10 out of 10 match. That's the best it can get. It doesn't get any better than that. Congratulations!"

By the end of Rachael's explanation, Nancy and I were jointly clutching a box of Kleenex. Our wait was over. The carefully avoided question of "What if there is no match?" could finally disappear from the far reaches of our minds—forever.

"Thank you, Rachael! Thank you from the bottom our hearts!"

"We'll talk later," she replied warmly.

Indeed, we would. A few days later, we were sitting in the University of Utah Transplant Unit with Rachael and her boss, Dr. Finn Bo Peterson.

The process has begun.

Summary: The transplant gods have given Nancy a fabulous welcome home present. The National Marrow Donor Program has identified a "10 out of 10" typed donor. A PERFECT match.

Huge love,

Winnie

The Many Kindnesses of Those around Us

September 30, 11:13 p.m.

Dear Friends and Family,

During our ordeal, we've been forced to make continual adjustments. Almost always, it's the result of something negative. The changes can be something big or small, like the unexpected lab value that once delayed our hospital discharge, or the very depressing revision to Nancy's initial diagnosis, or the constantly changing percentage concerning Nancy's survival.

We've learned to "roll with the punches."

We've had no choice.

After learning that leukemia specialist Dr. Fred Appelbaum could "fit us in as soon as we can get there," I called Atlantic Southeast Airlines (ASA) to see if Nancy might be eligible to fly on an employee pass to Seattle (even though she was on a medical leave of absence). When I reached her supervisor, Melodie, and explained our situation, she said, "I'll call you right back. I just need to check a few things with the head of HR."

In less than five minutes, Melodie called back: "Great news! ASA will give you and Nancy positive-space, round-trip, first-class passes. We're all rooting for Nancy."

"Positive space" meant we did not have to fly standby as is customary when flying on a pass. "First class" meant comfort. (This rare type of pass is usually reserved for senior executives of the company.) Essentially, ASA offered us free round-trip, first-class tickets to Seattle.

I was more than a little bit relieved. I had frequently worried about the toll the trip might have on Nancy, and this type of pass would make the trip light years easier for her than I had envisioned. I expressed my deepest thanks to Melodie and ASA. It's humbling to think that people at a large company like ASA, a Delta Airlines affiliate, would show such kindness.

But just a few hours later, I received an even more amazing call from Gil Williams, President of Royal Street Corporation, the parent company of the Deer Valley Resort, where I am the longtime medical director. "Winnie," he said, "Edgar and Polly want to fly you to Seattle on their plane. They don't want Nancy in an airport full of germs. They want the trip to be as easy as possible for her. When can you leave?"

I was so overwhelmed it took me a moment to respond. "Gil, are you sure? That seems like too much."

"I am sure. It's exactly what Edgar and Polly want for Nancy. Would it be better to leave from the Heber Airport or do you want to leave from the private airport next to Salt Lake International?"

As most of you know, Heber is a small private airport only twenty-five minutes away from Woodland. "I will check with Nancy, but Heber should work really well. Thanks, Gil. And please give Edgar and Polly our heartfelt thanks, too." Gil then unexpectedly added that Edgar and Polly hoped Nancy felt well enough to spend a few extra days in Seattle: "They've told their pilot to bring you home after you've had a few days to unwind."

Not surprisingly, it took an entire day to persuade Nancy to accept the Stern's kind and generous offer. She thought it far too extravagant, but Nancy finally agreed to make an exception. (I must admit I had to laugh to myself that it took Nancy so long to accept something so positive. But I did guess right: in the end, she decided on Heber.)

Summary: Nancy and I have made an "adjustment" to our Seattle trip plan. Instead of flying commercially, we will be flying in a private jet, an unbelievably generous gift from our friends Edgar and Polly Stern. We continue to be amazed by the kindness of those around us.

So much love,

Winnie

Free as a Bird

October 3, 1:32 a.m.

Dear Friends and Family,

Much of Nancy's adult life has revolved around airplanes.

During Nancy's thirty-three years as a flight attendant, she has flown on almost every type of commercial aircraft utilized in the United States. The exception would be the Concorde, though she did get to see one up close and personal at John F. Kennedy International Airport—better known as JFK. (She watched it take off and land.)

Until yesterday, Nancy's most memorable air travel experience was a trip from Salt Lake City to Yellowstone National Park in a T33 "Shooting Star," a World War II fighter jet restored and owned by a friend of mine, Dr. Bruce Huchinsen. Bruce used his jewel of an aircraft to commute between Utah and the Yellowstone National Park. The T33 is a two-seat airplane in which the pilot and passenger are beneath a glass bubble, sitting one behind the other. Nancy was strapped into the rear seat like a fighter copilot and had one of those black plastic devices that covered her mouth and nose and delivered oxygen during the flight. After the flight was completed, Bruce related to me the story of his new copilot Nancy breathing rapidly during the takeoff and the entire first part of the flight before adjusting to a normal breathing rate.

Nonetheless, as much as Nancy enjoyed her flight in a WWII vintage plane, there should be no doubt about how she would describe her all-time favorite flight if asked now. She would, without any hesitancy, talk about her experience yesterday.

Unlike most of our prior airplane trips, we were in no hurry to arrive at Heber Airport early. Departure time was "around

11 a.m.," and we were armed with the knowledge that the plane would not leave until we were safely on board. Once we were checked through the private gate at the airstrip, we drove right up to and then parked beside a Cessna Citation Jet whose call letters on the tail matched the numbers Gil had emailed me. Chief pilot Ed Dusang and his copilot Jeff Hansen greeted us as we got out of our car. Jeff wouldn't let me carry our bags, rather he grabbed them from our trunk and loaded them carefully into the plane's underbelly, while Ed helped us into the cabin of the four-passenger aircraft that would transport Nancy and me to Seattle.

After making sure we were comfortable, Ed served us drinks, showed us the emergency exit in the rear of the plane, tested our seat belts, and confirmed that our seats were upright. Only then did he return to the cockpit, where Jeff had finished his preflight checks and started both engines. Nancy grabbed my hand as we slowly taxied down the runway. Once we had been cleared for takeoff, Ed turned and gave us a thumbs-up through the open cockpit door.

Our takeoff acceleration was so rapid it felt as if we had been shot out of a cannon. We were airborne in seconds and circled momentarily above Heber before we headed northwest. The plane windows were surprisingly large and the view was spectacular, especially since the aspens and scrub oak displayed outsized patches of dark red and bright yellow below us. Excitedly, Nancy pointed and said, "Look, Winnie." I leaned toward her for a better view out the window on her side of the plane. I gazed as a familiar edifice, our home, disappeared below us as we rapidly winged our way toward our destination. In a minute or two, we were witnessing the exquisite beauty of Park City. Below us, the majesty of the peaks and ski slopes that make up the Deer Valley Resort slowly faded as we headed into the clouds and our ultimate cruising altitude of 36,000 feet.

In normal times, to experience a ride in a private jet is a thrill—in unusual times a godsend. The seats were large, covered in soft leather, and had controls for more adjustments than I knew what to do with without assistance. The cabin had room for all of our belongings, and the desk table could be utilized for eating, working, or playing games with other passengers. There were connections for all of our electronics, and the cockpit door remained open so we could watch as the pilots flipped switches, examined dials, and navigated the plane through the clouds. The box lunches Ed served us about a half hour into the flight had more food and snacks than we could eat and as much wine and soft drinks as we wanted to drink, responsibly. (We drank both.) And best of all, our pilots were gracious and kind, willing to answer all of our many questions about the aircraft. (They also were quick to point out any sights either of them deemed interesting.)

As I shared a moment ago, this isn't a time of normalcy.

At some point shortly after takeoff, I was struck by the thought that this could be Nancy's last trip. Ever. Consequently, I found myself preoccupied for much of the rest of our flight. My mind raced as it organized and reorganized the many topics I wanted to discuss with Dr. Appelbaum.

Nancy, on the other hand, soaked up every second of being far away from her medical nightmare. Her forehead lines were barely visible and her smile was relaxed and effortless. When I asked how she was feeling, she gazed out my window then looked me in the eye and responded, "I feel like I'm floating. I've been in the air so many times over the years, but it has never felt like this before. I feel as free as a bird. I don't want to ever land."

Nancy did sleep the last part of the trip, and I rubbed her hand that I had been holding the entire time. Only when Ed turned in the cockpit and said to me, "You might want to give her a nudge. Mt. Rainier is especially beautiful today," did Nancy awake up just in time to see us fly close enough that we could almost reach out and touch the snowcap that quickly drifted by our window.

The smoothness of our landing was as impressive as the acceleration of our original takeoff. As we pulled to a stop at our "parking space" at Boeing Field, Seattle's private airport, a black limousine appeared and parked directly next to the plane. As we exited, the driver loaded our bags.

In minutes, we were headed toward the Fred Hutchinson Cancer Center, where our next day's appointment loomed ahead of us. Our hotel was directly across the street from the center. There had been no long lines, no waiting for the counter personnel, no baggage checks or long walks through a busy terminal, and no shoe or belt removal. No one had stared at Nancy's semi-bald head wondering if it was a medical condition or a fashion statement. And most importantly, there were not many uninvited germs to test her impaired immunity.

Though Edgar and Polly were not with us on the plane to Seattle, we certainly felt their kindness and their love during the entire flight. Their feelings were reflected in Ed's last words as we exited the limo in front of our hotel: "Good luck tomorrow. Give me a call to let me know which day you want to go home. Remember what the Sterns said: 'No hurry.'"

Summary: Yesterday Nancy and I took a magical airplane ride to Seattle for our consultation. We are basking in the support of all of our friends and especially on this day, Edgar and Polly Stern.

With love,

Winnie

Nectar of the Gods

October 3, 9:28 p.m.

Dear Friends and Family,

"Well, Nancy, what do you think?"

"I think . . ." Nancy scratched the pretty pink hat covering her now fuzzy head, ". . . that I'm ready for a drink."

Nancy's full-throated laugh was bursting with mischief. It was not the laugh of someone in pain. And it wasn't the laugh of someone burdened by the specter of a terrible disease. Rather, it was a laugh brimming with joy and genuinely from the heart. It was the same laugh I first heard twenty-eight years ago on our very first date.

As I shared with you many letters ago, during the first few hours of my very first date with Nancy, we discussed religion, death, kids, and the meaning of life. But I must admit, after three hours of nonstop talking as we watched the sun slowly fade and dip behind the Absaroka Mountains that lined the horizon in the northern portion of Yellowstone National Park—we got thirsty. So we somewhat nervously headed to the *Two Bit Saloon* in Gardner, Montana, for a drink,

(There's something to be said about the "circle of life." In many ways it seems like we have come full circle. Today's laugh sounded just like our first time together. I loved that laugh then. And I still do now.)

Tonight, as we laughed together so many years later, we made our way to Joey's, an upscale bar and restaurant surrounded by a marina on the shore of Lake Union in Seattle, Washington. Outside the full-length tableside window were row after row of sailboats bobbing up and down like corks in the never-ending waves. Beyond the boats were seaplanes taking off and landing at regular five-minute intervals. And beyond the seaplanes was an endless horizon where the lake merged with the sky. It was a romantic spot, and I felt like a young lover as I gently held Nancy's hand and got lost in eyes that were even a deeper blue than the sky outside the restaurant's large bay window.

Joey's sits across the street from the Fred Hutchinson Cancer Center, next to our hotel. Today we obtained a second opinion from Dr. Fred Appelbaum, during more than an hour and a half of deliberations at the "Fred Hutch." A world-renowned expert in both transplantation and acute myeloid leukemia (AML), Dr. Appelbaum had been both scholarly and engaging. He told us ever so kindly, "I can easily picture my wife and me on your side of the table."

At the conclusion of our session, Nancy needed an escape from numbers and studies, treatments and side effects, and deliberations and decisions about her future. So I forced thoughts of Dr. Appelbaum out of my mind as I asked Sally, our waitress, "What would you suggest? This is a very special occasion for us."

"Our house specialty is a drink called a Bellini," she replied. "It is named after Giovanni Bellini, a famous painter during the Italian Renaissance. He created it in Italy in the 1930s." She pointed to a picture of the drink on the menu: "It is a frozen blend of sangria, rum, champagne, and peaches. It comes by the pitcher."

"I can't say that I'm familiar with the painter, but the drink sounds incredible," I replied. "We'll take a pitcher."

Our Bellinis arrived almost too picturesque to drink, a tall, elegant carafe displaying layers of red-and-orange swirls, with peaches floating on top as highlights. Sally gave the contents a hard stir and the colored layers suddenly transformed into a bright-purple slurry. She poured the almost luminous mixture into extra-large martini glasses and added a garnish of fresh pineapple, cherries, and limes. The drink's taste was matched only by the drink's beauty, and the pitcher was nearly empty before we began talking about our trip's "opportunities."

Nancy informed me she had made her first decision.

"Exciting news, Winnie. I feel really good and really strong today. Let's accept Edgar and Polly's offer and spend the next two days in Seattle."

Quite simply, we reveled in the possibilities of the next two days together.

The Space Needle.

Bainbridge Island.

Pike Place Market.

The many options were quickly listed on the back of a Joey's napkin next to an artist's rendering of Mr. "Bellini." We talked about fresh seafood for dinner and walks along the lake. A little overwhelmed, Nancy abruptly changed course: "I might just want to lie in bed and do nothing except watch sunsets."

"Whatever you want, my love. We're on our second honeymoon, aren't we?"

Indeed, our evening was reminiscent of the first night following our wedding when we spent an entire evening on a beach in Tahiti, toasting our marriage with a blend of juices and alcohol served in a single coconut with two straws.

Nancy and I clinked glasses to each potential activity and without expressing it, we also toasted our relief. The meeting that would shape our future together was finally behind us.

Nancy poured the last few Bellini ounces into my near-empty glass. I convinced her to put her straw in my glass and share the remaining "nectar from the gods." Effortlessly, with no change in her jovial presence, she took my hands so that all four of our hands rested next to the empty pitcher. "All right, Winnie. Let's figure this out. What do you think?"

I wanted to say, "Let's have another pitcher first." Instead, I replied softly, "Nancy, I will help analyze the information that we've been given and make lists of pros and cons. I'll do anything for you. But you're the decision maker for our treatment options."

"I know I am."

"So let's start with the transplant question."

"Dr. Appelbaum was really good, wasn't he?"

"Do you have any doubts about that choice?"

Dr. Appelbaum had been better than good. For almost two months, we have been trying to decide if a transplant was the superior route rather than undergoing two more rounds of chemotherapy. Every physician we polled used different numbers from different studies. Today, Dr. Appelbaum explained each of those studies, drew graphs on his whiteboard, and then individualized the data to Nancy.

He had started our meeting by saying, "The survival rate in Nancy's case with chemotherapy is only 25%, maybe as high as 27%. With a bone marrow transplant her survival chance jumps to 63%, though some of the survivors, maybe 10%, have quality of life issues due to graft-versus-host disease." Dr. Appelbaum went on to explain where the earlier 10–15% and 40% numbers had originated, and why neither applied to Nancy. His calm manner, confident deportment, and precise understanding of the known facts made the decision very clear.

"Nancy, I have no doubts. Transplant. Are you ready for it?"

"I am. I don't want to go through another round of chemotherapy waiting for the donor. What if the donor is in Iraq?"

"Then I'll fly to Baghdad. If he's on the space station, I'll go to the moon for you. It will be really hard to do another round of chemotherapy now that you've made the decision. I'll call Rachael at 8 a.m. tomorrow so we can move forward as quickly as possible."

"What about the type, Winnie? I really do need your help on that decision."

I needed help, too. Dr. Appelbaum favored Nancy having a "mini," but he had admitted during our meeting that the final data on that type of transplant was still a few years away. He felt confident the study he himself was conducting would conclude that the "mini" was just as effective as a "full" transplant but with less mortality and fewer side effects. But there were still a lot of unanswered questions.

Would his numbers change as the study progressed?

Would new or different side effects to the "mini" be discovered?

How should we decide between "experimental" versus "standard" therapies?

"I don't have a strong opinion yet, do you Nancy? I want to speak to Finn Bo on that one."

(Dr. Finn Bo Peterson, head of the transplant team at the University of Utah, has been leaning toward the full, myeloablative type of surgery. However, he freely admits the "full" transplant is more intense and much harder on the body.)

"Let's defer that one for now. Both Dr. Peterson and Dr. Appelbaum said we have plenty of time before we have to make that decision."

"Moving on, Winnie, I was really impressed with Dr. Appelbaum. Do you think we should do the transplant up here?"

I couldn't help but think to myself is this "southern speak?" Is Nancy really letting me know she wants her transplant in Seattle?

"There is no doubt moving to Seattle will present some logistical challenges. But I will figure out every detail if you want to come up here."

"But what about Jaret and Jayna? How would that work?"

"I don't know. But what I do know is that they want whatever is best for you."

Nancy sighed, and I noticed the first signs of melancholy. Her shoulders hunched forward a little and her eyes were not quite as wide as they had been earlier in the evening. "I want to make all of our decisions right now, Winnie. I'm tired of agonizing. But I guess we need to talk to Finn Bo first. I guess a couple more days is not the end of the world."

"No, it isn't. We're almost there. Let's go back to the room, rest a bit, and have an amazing dinner. As of right now, we're officially on a real vacation."

With only our water glasses, we toasted each other and to what lies ahead of us.

Summary: Our meeting with Dr. Fred Appelbaum, a world-renowned expert, was very productive and led to our first major decision. Nancy will proceed with a transplant. To celebrate our decision, we will stay a few days in Seattle to enjoy ourselves.

Much love,

Winnie

Another One Bites the Dust

October 6, 4:18 a.m.

Dear Friends and Family,

Nancy has made another critical and momentous decision that we want to share with you, but instead of starting my progress report abruptly—let me bring you up to date on other matters first. (I think when writers do this in their works of fiction or, for that matter, nonfiction this is called building the aura of suspense.) So let me begin our continuing story by sharing with you the outcome of our Seattle trip.

After two delightfully carefree days in Seattle during which we dined atop the Space Needle, visited the Seattle Art Museum, and shopped at the renowned Pike Place Market, Nancy and I boarded Polly and Edgar Stern's plane for a relaxing flight back to Utah. We are accustomed, as frequent standby passengers, to traveling light.

On our return trip, though, we were not flying standby. We had as much luggage space as we could ever want in this lifetime. So we took advantage of this once-in-a-lifetime opportunity to bring home a multicolored, uniquely shaped, hand-blown vase for our dining room table, as well as a huge cold "travel box" containing fresh salmon, oysters, mussels, and crab.

(While there are not sufficient words to express our gratitude to the Sterns for converting a stressful medical-related trip into an unanticipated glorious respite, I will say "thank you" once again. Thank you from the bottom of our hearts.)

Nancy and I came home completely refreshed and recharged, and we phoned Finn Bo (Dr. Peterson) as soon as we arrived in Woodland. For nearly an hour, Dr. Peterson answered our questions and then Nancy and I spent another hour or so in deliberation,

The next chapter in our journey may surprise you. Nancy has chosen a hospital room in Salt Lake City. After countless hours spent researching our options, it turns out that the survival rates for a transplant patient at the University of Washington in Seattle are essentially the same as the survival rates of patients at the University of Utah in Salt Lake City.

We were thoroughly impressed with Dr. Appelbaum, his program, and the facilities in Seattle, but when Nancy searched her soul deeply, she felt equally positive about Dr. Peterson and the program in Salt Lake City. Naturally, the crucial factor that served to tip the balance was Nancy's desire not to disrupt Jaret and Jayna's lives. Even though they have both stated unequivocally and without hesitation that they would relocate to Seattle, their mother did not want to disrupt their lives further.

So another major decision is now in the rearview mirror, but we still need to determine the type of transplant. Nancy has recently endured a long battery of tests to see if she is strong enough to attempt the full myeloablative transplant. If it is determined that she can't withstand the procedure, the choice will be made for us and she will have the "mini." While Nancy is chronologically older than anyone who has ever attempted the full transplant before, Finn Bo thinks she is in excellent shape for her age. He does, however, want a more detailed look at her heart, lungs, kidneys, and GI system. (He must have seen her doing laps in the hallway while having her chemotherapy.)

We are more than a little bit nervous to travel back into the world of needles and vital signs again. But Nancy seems at peace, in large measure from the support we have been given by so many of our friends. Thanks for your continued thoughts and prayers. They will, as they have in the past, help us prepare.

Summary: Nancy has decided to have her transplant in Utah. The only decision left is the type of transplant—mini versus full.

My sincerest thanks,

Winnie

Laughter Is the Best Medicine

October 9, 6:43 p.m.

Dear Friends and Family,

This afternoon, the phone was ringing like a siren's song as we opened the door when we returned from our brisk morning walk. After running into our well-lit kitchen to grab the phone, I saw the name on the caller ID. Instinctively I hesitated as I took a deep breath. Nancy looked at me with an unspoken alarm, silently asking, "What's the matter?"

"Dr. Winn, this is Rachael from the transplant team. I have exciting news. Your donor has consented to the transplant."

A single tear rolled down Nancy's cheek because I had been holding the phone so she could hear my conversation. Her tear matched mine. Another piece of the puzzle was now in place.

"Thank you so very much, Rachael."

Recently, our time at home has been pretty quiet and uneventful, so I haven't written as much to you. However, during this time away, we have made a "family" discovery. On the days when I'm not at the office early, Jayna doesn't have school, and Nancy is not hurrying to a doctor's appointment or pre-transplant test, our family has rediscovered a special time—breakfast.

With everyone rested, each of us now takes turns cooking and serving the first meal of the day. It's quickly becoming a family tradition. Nancy's taste buds have rallied from the burn of chemotherapy and she craves Krispy Kreme donuts. So I serve her two KKs—one glazed and one chocolate. (Why not? In a little more than a week, Nancy is due for her next round in the hospital. She won't be eating much then, if at all.)

Food is merely a small part of our new ritual. Breakfast often extends to midday. Whether we're relaxing in the dining room or lounging on our new living room furniture, we share family memories, tell personal stories, read the many cards from friends and acquaintances, and look at almost any type (regardless of subject) of interesting pictures, particularly of faraway places and lands.

Not surprising, the fall sunshine comes from a lower point on the horizon each day now, but it still catches the leaves on the many aspens and cottonwoods. The trees shimmer in the soft breeze and shine with such a brilliant gold they seem ready to burst and explode into a million pieces of dazzling rubies, sapphires, and diamonds.

Quite simply, we feel rich both in spirit and in our souls. We are very fortunate to have each other—our little family.

We love our homey paradise by the river.

We love that Nancy is home and feeling decent.

We love that she is getting strong.

And most of all, we love that she is getting ready for what lies ahead.

On most days, we take turns playing music on the stereo system, we go to almost any movie matinee that appeals to Nancy, and we play Monopoly, Clue, and computer games until far too late in the evening. We also (far too often) fall asleep watching videos—all three of us (Nancy, Jayna, and me) in our king-size bed. Unfortunately, Jaret's school schedule makes him a weekend-only visitor. But on the many frequent weekends he is with us, he stakes out his favorite spot—on the floor surrounded by lots and lots of pillows and blankets.

Occasionally, we visit a restaurant that strikes Nancy's fancy. Most often, though, we dine on delicious meals that are silently dropped off on our doorstep by the informal network of supporters. (We feel your love, and the food that you provide us nourishes not only our bodies, but it strengthens our souls as well.)

Our home also continues to be filled with something that similarly sustains our journey—laughter. It is more important now than in the past. Laughter soothes our family's collective soul.

"Look, Dad. Mom has a natural Mohawk."

With great hesitancy, Nancy now allows Jayna and me to examine her "fuzzy" head from all sides. Nancy's salt-and-pepper strands, now barely an inch long, come together like small tee-pees in the center of her scalp, extending from the cowlick in the front of her head to the endearing singular mole toward the back.

(Jayna's right. It does look like a Mohawk.)

As you also know, an important part of my morning ritual is kissing Nancy's head. I perform this simple ceremony each and every day—right after Nancy has her second donut and before we do the dishes.

"Your turn to cook, Dad. And to do the dishes."

"Why are you so mean to me, Jayna?"

"You know, Dad."

"What, sweetheart?"

"I would definitely treat you better if you had leukemia like Mom."

Jayna's deadpanned statement is, as always, timed perfectly. It makes all three of us laugh. Especially Nancy.

Summary: Our time together at home has been magnificent.

Sent with love,

Winnie

When Final Really Is Final

October 10, 11:33 p.m.

Dear Friends and Family,

Yesterday I wrote you about our fun-filled time at home.
(That was yesterday.)
Today began something like this:
"Good morning, sweetheart. How was your night?"
"You were asleep the minute you hit the pillow, Winnie."
Uh-oh.
Once again, my bride's southern roots were in full display.
She avoided my question.
"I know, Nancy. I was exhausted. Chuck and I rode hard after work. And the clinic was way too busy for a fall day. But what about you? Did your leg bother you?"
Nancy's sciatica has been a nagging issue since her last hospitalization when she overdid her exercise. (She's not allowed to take anti-inflammatory drugs because of her blood-thinning medicine.)
"It did ache last night. So I took a pain pill. That helped. But . . ."
Nancy didn't have to finish the sentence. I recognized the look on her face. She's having difficulty sleeping for the same reason I am—we're both thinking about the decision.
As we wait for the final word from the hospital that our "angel" donor is medically fit and willing to share his precious bone marrow, it isn't difficult to be constantly (and rightly so) preoccupied. Nancy and I both find ourselves continually ruminating over the sound bites we've heard from experts in the field of leukemia. We've found many hematologists and

oncologists willing to discuss Nancy's case, but their voices reflect the uncertainty of current knowledge.

The day after one prominent doctor made the statement, "I see no reason for Nancy to attempt an unmatched Allo (or full transplant). It's too risky," another specialist summed up his opinion with, "A standard full transplant gives Nancy the best chance of a durable remission (or cure)."

Other calls I have made have ended with, "There is no wrong answer or choice in Nancy's case" or "At our center, we'd consider an autologous transplant." (An option that has never even appeared on our radar screen.)

We have been told so many conflicting things by so many well-meaning experts:

"Chemotherapy alone might be the best way to go."

"A mini has the same numbers but with far less toxicity. The full transplant has a 20–30% mortality rate in the first month."

"The study using the mini has only twenty-five subjects. It is a very small study."

"The full transplant has been around for years. The study comparing it to the mini isn't finished. It won't be done for another couple of years."

The single insight that has helped us more than any other to get through the complex and sometimes conflicting studies and statistics is something our doctor Finn Bo told us: "You can change your mind up until the first day of the 'conditioning' regimen of medicines that will ablate your bone marrow. Once that starts, there's no turning back."

"Was your mind racing again, Nancy?"

"Yes, one minute I think I want the mini, the next the full."

"What do you think, Winnie?"

What do I think?

I think I'm scared and sad. I am extremely sad. I think I want to scream. I want to stop thinking. (What I really want to know is what Nancy is thinking about in the middle of the night, in the darkness.)

What I am thinking is, "How can I help?"

"Nancy, I think that whatever you decide, we'll be all right. I think—no, I know—that you are really physically and mentally strong now. I'll be holding your hand the whole way. And you have so many people rooting for you."

"Will you make breakfast today, Winnie?"

Summary: We are wading through the various transplant alternatives. There are many divergent opinions among the experts as Nancy's transplant date comes ever closer.

Fondly,

Winnie

Merriment in a Dark Time

October 14, 2:20 a.m.

Dear Friends and Family,

The last three weeks have been glorious.

Quite simply, we have watched the leaves change while waiting for our lives to change, as well.

Yesterday, Wednesday, October 13, was Decision Day.

Yesterday Nancy and I had an hour-and-a-half meeting with the transplant team at the University of Utah. After our meeting had ended and as we were walking down the hall toward the fifth floor elevator, I took Nancy's hand in mine after looking at her face, "You look a little blue, darlin'. What did you think?"

Nancy squeezed back tightly. "I'm still happy with our decision. I just wish I could've closed my ears after the first twenty minutes."

I couldn't have agreed any more with Nancy. The first twenty minutes of our meeting were great. Dr. Tsai, Dr. Peterson's partner on the transplant team, had expertly explained his views on the mini versus full transplant dilemma. He was clear, concise, and straightforward. Dr. Tsai had been the best yet at explaining both the pros and the cons. Those twenty minutes were just what we needed to finally make our choice.

After that?

The meeting was a complete nightmare. I should have brought earplugs for Nancy. She was forced to sit quietly and listen about the seemingly endless list of awful things that might happen to her during and after her transplant.

We learned the side effects of each poison medicine Nancy will receive.

We explored how and why any of her organs can fail.

We discussed scientifically why the next thirty, or even one hundred, days might be a living hell.

The descriptions of potential side effects went on and on.

As a medical professional, I understand the concept of informed consent.

Simply, we were not prepared for *"Sign here, Nancy, that you may live. But it might be hell. Or, as I've made you acutely aware, sign below that you fully realize that if you don't experience a living hell, you might simply die."*

I was more than a little surprised that Dr. Tsai didn't ask, "How much do you want to hear, Nancy?" All along, Nancy has only wanted information when she was ready. Her beautiful face is so easy to read. Couldn't Dr. Tsai see the look in her eyes? Every line on her face said, "Not now."

We had been sent a consent form to review before the meeting. It was twenty-six single-spaced pages. Twenty-six pages. I'd read every line, crying by the end of each section. When I gave Nancy the option of hearing a three-word summary, she gladly agreed. She quickly signed the last page; not reading a word, as I chose my three words carefully, "Transplants are dangerous."

She was able to quip, "Let me guess. It says I have a 50% chance of dying. And if I don't die, everything that can go wrong will go wrong with any part of my body at any time."

(Maybe she had read the consent form.)

All I could think about were two things: Why hadn't I brought earplugs for her? And how can I save her from the heartache I am feeling?

Jayna, who had also attended the meeting, looked at Nancy and me. As usual, she initiated the positive words we needed for the moment. "I think it's amazing that Mom will have a new blood type," she said as she placed a sweet kiss on Nancy's cheek. "You'll be A-positive. And the nurse told me you'll get the color of the donor's hair. You'll have more fun as a blonde, don't you think, Mommer?"

Nancy whispered, "I'll be glad just to have hair again."

"Maybe we should think of this hospitalization as a test, Nancy. And Dr. Tsai said you will assume the donor's A-positive blood type," I added. I took a pen out of my pocket as well as the card Dr. Tsai had given me. I wrote the letter A and next to it the symbol + on the back of the card for Nancy and Jayna to see.

"Can't do any better than an A-plus."

(My one-liners are nowhere near as funny as Jayna's or Nancy's.)

"How 'bout you, Jayna? Comfortable with Mom's decision?"

"Totally, Dadder. I was leaning in that direction all along. Dr. Tsai merely sealed the deal. And Jaret told me last night he felt the same way. He's confident you're going to sail through this, Mommer. Me, too."

Nancy turned toward me, "Winnie, your turn. Did we make the right decision?"

"I . . ."

I was saved by the opening of the elevator door, as a family of four and a family of three entered the cab, squeezing Nancy, Jayna, and me to the back. Nancy raised her index finger to her lips. No need to answer my question, her gesture told me. She knew my answer anyway.

Nancy squeezed my hand again and winked. The father next to me smiled.

Once again, our family found merriment in a dark time.

Summary: Even though only Nancy's vote counted, our family unanimously decided that she should have the full (traditional) transplant. I will send details of the next part of our journey later this evening when everyone is in bed.

Love,

Winnie

A Journey of Daydreams

October 14, 10:11 p.m.

Dear Friends and Family,

We are home now and everyone is tucked safely between the sheets. So I want to explain to you what will happen in the ensuing days, weeks, and months ahead.

Nancy will enter the University of Utah Hospital in three days, October 17. Once there, she will receive six days of toxic chemotherapy. The panel of drugs will completely obliterate her bone marrow over a nine-day period. By far, this upcoming period will be the most intense (and therefore toxic) chemotherapy Nancy has received since May. And this phase is called "conditioning therapy." The drugs are meant to totally destroy her existing bone marrow cells, thereby setting the "conditions" for her new bone marrow cells. In theory (and hopefully in practice), this therapy will destroy every cell of her existing and potentially leukemia-harboring bone marrow tissue.

After the next ten day's chemotherapy ordeal, she will receive her MUD (matched unrelated donor) transplant. Many of you have asked if a bone marrow transplant is an actual operation. It is not. Rather than an actual surgery, Nancy will receive her new bone marrow cells via an IV catheter that enters a large vein in her chest, just like any other medicine or the many blood and blood product transfusions she has received in past months. Quite miraculously, the special donor bone marrow cells will know where to look for a "new home" outside of Nancy's bloodstream.

Once inside Nancy's bones, we will need to wait for an "engraftment." This is where the donor's bone marrow cells will, with any luck, replace Nancy's natural bone marrow tissue that should have been "destroyed" by the potent chemotherapy. During this period, once again, Nancy is at great risk for unusual "opportunistic" infections as well as bleeding.

At this point, Nancy will have zero natural immunity, zero natural ability to clot her blood, and zero ability to make her own oxygen-carrying red blood cells. She will survive on blood and blood product transfusions for up to three weeks. The earliest Nancy might be able to leave the hospital is four weeks after her transplant, though six weeks is probably more realistic (and only then if there are no complications). We've been quoted a 20% death rate during this first, critical phase.

When Nancy leaves the hospital, she will move to an apartment that we've rented in the Sugar House area of Salt Lake City, about eight minutes from the University of Utah Hospital. Our transplant "contract" requires us to stay close to the hospital for a minimum of three months because the critical landmark of success is one hundred days post-transplant.

The major worry during this "out of the hospital" post-transplant period is something called "graft-versus-host" disease, a condition where the donor graft attacks the body it has entered after the transplant. During these three months, we will be monitored very closely with frequent outpatient visits to the Blood and Marrow Transplant Clinic (BMT Clinic). On the day of our recent orientation meeting, we visited the BMT Clinic and witnessed a lot of bald folks wearing specialized masks to avoid infection. (At this point, we can't wait until Nancy has her very own anti-infection mask.)

So that's the summary for the next leg of our journey. Not surprisingly, we have no doubt it will be a very long and very difficult road to travel. But Nancy, as best as I can tell, seems prepared for what lies ahead.

As I turn to look at her now as she slumbers beside me, I observe a whisper of contentment on her lips that shape a faint grin. I wonder if she is dreaming of her eventual return to our comfortable bed, her health fully restored?

I dream too, but my dreams are "day" dreams. (I am experiencing a nervous period where I have great difficulty sleeping, so I daydream instead and try to picture her prospects the way I want them to be.)

We are about to take a very big risk.

We hope to win big.

But today, the mountain seems steep and the climb very long.

I can't yet see the top.

When I "dream," I force myself to imagine snowflakes lightly floating outside our Woodland home's bedroom windows, covering the trees' bare branches like the softest and fluffiest of frosting. I gaze at Nancy beside me and concentrate on how it will feel to share a white winter wonderland when she comes home to the bed in which she now lies. At best, it will be a long time from today.

As I've said to you before, I've never much been one to anticipate my next day off, my next vacation, or even my next special event. Living in such a wonderful place as we do, I've been too busy enjoying the present to anticipate the future. Not today. It is a different chapter in my life. I want the next one hundred days to pass like a quiet storm in the late evening. I want to wake up from my "dream" to bright daylight as if nothing happened during the dark hours of night.

The address of our new home will be: Nancy Winn, Patient Extraordinaire, 5th Floor (I'll send the exact room at some point), University of Utah Hospital, 50 North Medical Drive, Salt Lake City, Utah, 84132.

P.S. We will be unable to find out much about Nancy's donor for one year. As part of the donor-recipient agreement we signed with the National Marrow Donor Program (NMDP), we are limited in finding out more about her donor. Likewise, he knows little about Nancy. With mortality rates so high, the NMDP feels it is best to reveal only the most basic information to either party.

But we do know this: The NMDP did reveal that the donor is a male, with A-positive blood type. Thankfully, we know he consented to give us his stem cells removed directly from his bone marrow. We asked for this method because this technique of collection carries a lower likelihood of graft-versus-host disease.

Without doubt, it is crystal clear to us that Nancy's donor is truly our "angel." Please send him your extra positive thoughts, appreciation, and gratitude.

Summary: Nancy begins her ablative chemotherapy in four days, and (if all goes well) we will reside in the hospital for four to six weeks and then live near the hospital in Salt Lake City for three months before returning home.

With love,

Winnie

The Last Supper

October 17, 8:44 p.m.

Dear Friends and Family,

Last night, the entire family ate our last dinner at the Market Street Grille, a Salt Lake City seafood eatery that is one of Nancy's favorites. We thoroughly enjoyed every bite. Nancy savored the Chilean Sea Bass she ordered, Jayna inhaled a huge plate of fried oysters, and I ate the Outer Banks Sea Scallops. Jaret, who doesn't like seafood, ate several loaves of bread and found a pasta dish he could devour that was devoid of fish.

As we sat together at dinner, we shared the unspoken knowledge that it would be a very long time before we would eat together again as a family. Surprisingly, Nancy celebrated with an inexpensive glass of "house" Sauvignon Blanc, stating, "My taste buds still aren't recovered enough to order a lavish 'vintage' wine." Even so, we still clinked glasses numerous times as each of us told and retold stories. All in all, it was an entirely relaxed and peaceful evening. On this bittersweet night, as each of us harbored unspoken fearful thoughts and unspoken feelings of melancholy, Nancy's wine glass was never half empty. Rather, it was always half full.

After leaving the restaurant, Jaret returned to Westminster College, while Jayna, Nancy, and I slept in the recently rented Salt Lake City apartment located in the Sugar House area of Salt Lake City. From there, it's an easy eight-minute drive to the University Hospital. (We have leased the apartment because Nancy is required to live close to the hospital once she is discharged after her transplant. We don't know exactly when that will occur until she is released. So we want to be sure we have secured housing for that much-anticipated event.)

Unexpectedly this morning, I awoke feeling like a night hob-goblin had beaten me with a sledgehammer. Every bone in my body ached, and each time I stretched out, another area of discomfort was revealed. I don't know if I slept poorly on the new bed or if I consumed too much wine. In reality it doesn't matter, though. There is only one thing on my mind: *What is Nancy feeling?*

I was stunned when Nancy greeted me with, "I don't want to go, Winnie," instead of her typical "Good morning." But before I could dislodge the too-large grapefruit that was in my throat, she added, "Just kidding. You take the first shower." Her face looked calm and her smile genuine.

When I returned a few minutes later, still dripping beneath my towel from my quick shower, I was expecting Nancy to be savoring her last moments between the sheets. Or quietly meditating in the living room. Or gazing out the window to catch a last glimpse of normalcy—the people, trees, and birds she might not view again for an eternity. But no, she was doing none of these things.

Nancy was making the bed.

As usual, she read my expression: "I want to leave it nice for Jayna. She'll be keeping this bed warm for me until I get out." (Though Nancy and I have urged Jayna to return to Vassar for her senior year of college, she will hear nothing of it.)

"I want to stay with you, Mommer," she told Nancy.

Similarly, she told me, "You'll need my help."

(It turns out that our new apartment will have an additional function—Jayna's classes at the University of Utah are going to be only minutes from the hospital. It seems that Nancy's "recovery" apartment is also going to be Jayna's "dorm.")

In the car on the way to the hospital, Nancy reiterated, "You know my only worry?"

I do know.

It's not pain.

It's not fear.

It's not uncertainty.

For what seemed like the thousandth time, she earnestly and matter-of-factly said, "I need to know that Jayna, Jaret, and you will be all right. If things don't go well, I need to know that you will take care of them. And that you will look for happiness wherever and with whomever without the memory of me holding you back."

"What about you, Nancy? Aren't you scared?"

Silence blanketed the car.

"A little, Winnie. But not as much as you."

The soft kiss Nancy placed on my cheek was especially warm today. And I found comfort, strength, and courage in her concern and love for our children and me.

Summary: Today Nancy entered the hospital for her transplant. It is hard to believe this day has arrived. She seems prepared.

All my love,

Winnie

The Transplant Shuffle

October 18, 8:02 p.m.

Dear Friends and Family,

Day one of Nancy's "ablative" chemotherapy is, in reality, day two of this hospitalization.

Nancy's body is experiencing a new drug named Busulfan, an especially toxic poison. As the strongest chemotherapy drug currently available, it has a singular purpose: it must totally obliterate Nancy's natural bone marrow, thereby ridding her body of any residual leukemia. (Consequently, I'm only going to work three days during these first two weeks.)

Today, as I headed to Salt Lake City after a full day of seeing patients at the office, I felt absolutely and completely sick to my stomach. By the time I would arrive, Nancy would be finishing her third dose of Busulfan. I didn't know what to expect, and I'd read and heard about all the negative possibilities.

Would I find Nancy wrenching continuously?

Would her mouth be full of sores?

Or worse yet, would her liver, kidney, or heart be showing potential devastating side effects?

Leukemia is a psychologically rough cancer. Whenever a leukemia patient achieves a remission, the patient feels nearly normal. But feeling normal makes it harder to face an uncertain future, particularly when it can mean a return to truly difficult times.

When I saw Nancy yesterday, she was in the middle of her third remission. She was feeling good. She was feeling strong. Her fuzzy head is the only thing that reminds her that she has a life-threatening disease—that and the elevator ride to the top floor of the hospital that also reminded her that she was once again going to be on the "floor nearest to heaven."

To my surprise as I entered "heaven," joyfulness filled the room. Jayna was taking a movie of her "Moo."

"Dad, come dance with Moo. She's doing the transplant shuffle."

For several minutes, Nancy and I "twisted and turned" just like Chubby Checkers. We kissed once and then we kissed again, Jayna recording it for posterity. It was magnificent and, at least for the moment, Nancy is doing fine.

Summary: We have survived the initial first two days in the hospital and Nancy's first day of toxic medicines. We danced and Nancy has promised that if she makes it through our ordeal, she will reprise her ballerina role in our new original staging of the ballet, Transplantland.

All my love,

Winnie

Luck Is Believing You're Lucky

October 19, 9:57 a.m.

Dear Friends and Family,

In just a few days, we have settled into Room 507 at the University of Utah Hospital—yet another new home.

Our room is probably a full third larger than the other various rooms on the cancer floor at LDS Hospital. Significantly, the bathroom is bigger and the closet space is increased dramatically. We now have a mammoth corkboard for pictures, more wall area for decorations, and there is space for not only the rollaway bed but two more chairs.

We are lucky. To have such a spacious room is really opportune. From what the nurses tell us, we'll reside here a lot longer than our current record of thirty-nine days, spent in Room 842 at LDS Hospital. (We can use every inch of living area. I suspect there will be nights when the whole family may "sleep over" to support Nancy during her most difficult challenges ahead.)

The best part, however, is not the room.

Rather, it is the fabulous view.

The entire outward-facing wall of our room is comprised of glass. Situated at the top of the east "bench" of the Wasatch Mountains, the University of Utah Hospital overlooks the entire Salt Lake Valley. About ten miles to the west, the barren Oquirrh Mountains jut upward, while to the northwest, the Great Salt Lake extends to the horizon. During the day, it is easy to identify the Mormon Tabernacle, the LDS Church Office Building, the Key Bank building, and other Salt Lake City landmarks. The sunsets are spectacular, and at night the city lights twinkle as far as the eye can see.

If you can believe it, we even have a remote control to close and open the blinds. For now, though, I only open the blinds briefly when Nancy is in her deepest sleep. Otherwise the blinds remain mostly closed. Not surprising, Nancy is focused inward and the beauty outside our room is a distraction. (I long for the day when I hear, *Winnie, what in the world is going on out there? Let's open the blinds.* But now is not the time for any distractions, no matter how beautiful.)

Nancy has been visiting "Dreamland" for the last two hours.

Me?

I've spent the entire time toying with our room number, Room 507.

Five plus zero plus seven equals twelve.

Twelve has never been lucky for me. If only we were in Room 508; the addition of the room numbers would equal thirteen, my basketball number in seventh grade. The pinnacle of my athletic pursuits, when I was a starting point guard in junior high school and we won our local tournament. But twelve? I have never received a dozen roses. The number twelve just doesn't do it for me.

Then I decide to look at each number individually.

Five. I love the number five.

Five is one of my favorite ages, when a child is just starting kindergarten.

A five-year-old child is not too shy to give me a hug.

A five-year-old child will gladly sit on their mom's or dad's lap during my exam.

Five. Now that's a great number.

What about seven?

A traditionally lucky number, seven is definitely lucky for me, especially now.

Why?

Nancy's birth month is July, the seventh month.

Nancy is definitely tied to the number seven. (It just can't get luckier than that.)

And zero?

That's easy. It's the answer to the question now defining our lives: "What happens if Nancy makes it through the next one hundred days?"

The lucky answer?
"Zero leukemia."
Room FIVE-ZERO-SEVEN.
A room virtually overflowing with luck.
Enough luck to share with our neighbors.
Enough luck for the whole bone marrow floor.
I need us to be in a lucky room. (We obviously are.)
Suddenly, I sense that Nancy is awake and I look into her sky-blue eyes: "What?" Nancy blinks three times in rapid succession, adjusting to the bright light in Room 507, "Did I fall asleep in the middle of my sentence or yours?"

"Neither, love. You finished your sentence right after reminiscing about how expressive Jayna's face was as a baby. Then, I'm sorry to report, you began snoring loud enough to wake up all the patients in the whole hospital. You were really in a deep sleep. I'm sorry if I woke you up just now."

"It's all right." Nancy opened her eyes wider, trying to better focus on the large, round wall clock opposite her bed. Despite two full days of poison flowing into her veins, Nancy's eyes still retain their spark and their exquisite beauty. (I could look at those eyes for an eternity, but I will gladly settle for another twenty years.)

"Is it eight o'clock already?"
"I really did sleep, didn't I?"
"I'm not throwing up yet."
"My mouth feels funny."
"I have a metallic taste in my mouth."
"I don't feel as bad as I thought I would today."
"What have you been doing?"
"Why such a big grin?"
"Am I getting that rash again?"
No you aren't, Nancy, I thought to myself. The total body, intensely itchy, reddish-orange rash that you developed yesterday is at bay for now. Fortunately, it was an insignificant, though annoying, side effect of the mouth ulcer medicine you took prior to beginning the new drugs. The rash is far more benign than the painful ulcers on the inside of your mouth that could be the potential entry point for a life-threatening germ. Thankfully the rash disappeared as rapidly as it covered your entire body once you finished your medicine.

After gathering her senses, I proudly related my "room number" game to Nancy, proclaiming, "We're very lucky to be in Room 507."

"I'm glad you think this room is lucky, Winnie. I've been worried. The sudden way we moved in made me think the last patient died here. I've tried not to think about it, but it's been a little frightening."

When we first arrived at the hospital two days ago, we were initially placed in Room 514, an "overflow" room just outside the Bone Marrow Unit. We were told the floor was full and that we would transfer into our permanent room in a few days.

Undeterred, I didn't change our "moving-in" routine. I spent a full forty-five minutes decorating our room. I placed our plastic flowers in all the unusual corners and shelves, hung the hand-carved birds that my partner Bob Evers created from exotic woods, and found a special place for each of Nancy's handpicked pictures.

As a result, the "white sterile box" was transformed into Nancy's personal hideaway. However, just as I received Nancy's final approval of my decorating efforts, our nurse, Gwen, entered the room and raised her eyebrows somewhat in shock: "Wow, you certainly didn't waste any time in making this room homey. But I was just told that Room 507 is available. It's directly across from the Bone Marrow Unit nursing station. It's opened up and we need to move you. I'm sorry you went to all this trouble, but 507 is a really nice room. It's one of my favorites."

"Don't be frightened, Nancy. I know this is a lucky room."

How could my numbers game have gone so wrong?

"Honey, I'll be right back. I need to make a bathroom run."

I have never lied to Nancy before, and I considered this only a slight "fib." I simply didn't want her to see my disappointment. But I must admit, I couldn't help but wonder if Room 507 might be bad luck?

I did make the trek to the bathroom, but my real purpose had nothing to do with my bladder. I actually needed to corner our nurse for this shift, Connie. Her last words when I met her were, "Please feel free to ask me any question."

"Connie, you may not be able to answer my question, but did the patient who was in our room before Nancy die?"

My question wasn't totally off the wall. Nancy had been quoted a 20–30% chance of not walking out of "that" room, and I simply needed to know the answer—for me and for Nancy. Before I could completely finish my question, though, Connie responded, "Heavens no. The previous patient went home earlier than we expected. The doctors sometimes fool us that way." Connie touched my shoulder as she handed me a Kleenex, "Don't worry, Winnie. You're in a good room. I know it. Nancy is doing great."

Events are already starting to blur for us—after only two days. We constantly watch staff scurry in and out through our always-closed door. They administer an endless supply of medicines, fluids, and treatments. Most of the time, Nancy's eyelids appear heavily weighed. She does her best to swish and spit four times a day to keep her mouth healthy. She blows into a bottle to help keep her lungs expanded.

I have always been good at remembering names, but I am beginning to wonder with each passing day.

Is our recreational therapist named Joanne?

Or is Joanne the nutritionist?

Maybe Joanne is the social worker?

How about the physical therapist?

Is Joanne the cute environmental health worker? (No, I actually do recall that her name is Juana. She is from Peru. The other day she and Jayna spoke Spanish for twenty minutes and formed an instant bond. Our room stays really clean.)

"Guess what, Nancy? I just spoke with Connie. She had very good news. The last patient in this room . . ."

Summary: Our new room is "The Lucky Room," FIVE-ZERO-SEVEN, University of Utah Hospital, 50 North Medical Drive, Salt Lake City, Utah 84132.

With luck,

Winnie

Pleasant Dreams, Sweetheart

October 24, 6:45 p.m.

Dear Friends and Family,

With only two more days left in her multiple drug pre-transplant chemotherapy regimen, Nancy is poised to begin a new drug, Cytoxan. Our nurse, Erlene, described Nancy's final "poison" as she hung the bag. As I listened, I couldn't help but wonder, "Why would a drug company include 'toxin' in a drug's name even though it ended with an 'a' not an 'i'?"

"Nancy, this medicine will make you pretty nauseated. It's noxious to the bladder, so we'll give you lots of fluid to minimize its effects. You will need to get up and go to the bathroom at least every hour. And Cytoxan sometimes burns on its way into your vein. Don't be afraid to ask for your pain meds. It's also not uncommon to have jaw pain and flushing and other side effects."

Nancy's expression to this warning was stoic and full of resolve. So when Jayna arrived to cover my absence, I left for work at the clinic with somewhat guarded confidence. Unfortunately, I found a much different Nancy when I returned to the hospital in the early evening. She was no longer the sleepy, mildly uncomfortable, slightly nauseated patient I left earlier. Instead, Nancy was tossing and turning in her bed. She struggled to say hello when she finally noticed me. As I looked at her face, I saw dry and peeling lips. Tense muscles furrowed her brow. After the hello and a noble attempt to smile, Nancy vomited.

Cytoxan.

Two doses.

One today, almost finished.

One tomorrow.

I cleaned up the floor next to Nancy's bed and went to the ice machine in the hall in anticipation of Nancy needing cold fluid. When I returned, I stroked her forehead and massaged her feet. Erlene brought Nancy a parade of drugs for nausea and pain. "Would you like a movie as a distraction?" I asked. Nancy didn't have the strength to speak, and I could sense that every bone in her body was aching, but she did nod her head. She even attempted to grin as she tried to make me feel better.

Upon finishing Nancy's foot massage, I heard the repetitive sound of restful breathing. It was followed by what has become one of my favorite sounds, Nancy's telltale snort. Finally, she was asleep. *Dances with Wolves* stayed in its package. There would not be any dancing for Nancy on this particular night.

Jayna, who left when I arrived, returned three hours later. She brought hugs, kisses, and her upbeat presence. Erlene came and removed the empty Cytoxan bag. Round one was in the history books.

Jayna's kiss, placed gently on her mom's fuzzy head, triggered open eyes, both wide and bright. "I'm cold," she said, after grabbing Jayna's hand.

I jumped immediately from my chair, a soft hospital blanket in hand.

"What will I ever do at home?"

"What's going to happen when I mention something and nobody responds?"

"Do you think I'm spoiled?"

Nancy giggled softly at her discomfort and went on to say, "The hospital stuff isn't so bad, Jayna."

"I sleep all day."

"I wake up and get nausea pills."

"I eat."

"I go back to sleep."

"I even had a funny dream while receiving this latest medicine."

"What's its name?"

"Oh, it doesn't matter . . ."

"What happened in the dream, Mommer?"

"Do you see that giant IV bag?"

"Which one, Mommer?"

"The one that looks like a cow's udder filled with milk?"

Since Nancy now battles constant nausea and her gastrointestinal lining is irritated as a result of her medicines, her oral intake has dropped to near zero. The "milk" bag she pointed to was actually filled with TPN, an abbreviation for total parenteral nutrition. We have been told Nancy won't be eating much the next couple weeks, so this liquid food will run day and night. Each bag of TPN was at least five times as big as the four others hanging from Nancy's IV pole. (Quite comically, it looks like milk going directly into Nancy's vein instead of being clear like water as in the other IVs.)

"I dreamed I was lying right here in bed, looking up at that ridiculous IV pole. I tried to read the names of the medicines on each of the three IV bags and the two IV bottles hanging from the pole. I asked the male nurse, who looked like Seth Meyers, 'Why are you giving me milk from a bag that is so much larger than the others?' But guess what? The reason the nurse looked like Seth Meyers is that I was actually part of a skit for *Saturday Night Live*. So the Seth Meyer look-alike flipped a switch on the IV pole and the bags and bottles begin to spin like a teacup ride at the circus and then smash, that big one with the white liquid food fell onto my face and smothered me."

"Pleasant dream, Mom. I like the South Sea Island one better."

"But Jayna, don't you realize the dream was good news? It meant I don't have to receive tomorrow's dose of that medicine. I remember its name now, too. Cytoxan."

In actuality, none of the six different IVs hanging from Nancy's pole fell onto her that night. She endured her last Cytoxan dose, still more than a bit stoic and resolved. She ached and she vomited and she made her hourly trips to the bathroom. And when the drugs were all finished—she went from feeling horrible to "not so bad." As she began to feel better, her first thought was "Where is the remote for the blinds? I bet it will be a pretty sunset tonight."

The sunset was certainly beautiful. As the Oquirrh Mountains on the horizon swallowed the bright-yellow orb, we watched red-and-orange cloud wisps fade slowly into gray as the darkness turned the city's buildings into dark shadows only visible due to the lights in the streets and in the windows of homes far below us.

"Another day comes to an end," I whispered to Jayna. With Nancy deciding to look outside for the first time of this hospitalization, the day held additional significance.

Nancy startled me when she raised her thumb to the air:

"And another treatment comes to an end."

"I am done."

"No more chemotherapy."

"I get to rest tomorrow."

"Then my transplant."

"Come give me a hug."

"Both of you."

Summary: A momentous day. Nancy finished her last "poison" medicine today. Chemotherapy will soon be an unpleasant, distant memory. She didn't experience any horrible, life-threatening side effects, though she did feel terribly sick with nausea and vomiting. After another day's rest, she will receive her transplant. Finally.

So much love,

Winnie

From This Day Forward

October 27, 5:32 a.m.

Dear Friends and Family,

"What's a bone marrow transplant procedure like?"
It's a frequent question.
So here's my attempt to describe it to you.
The two lab technicians were all grins when they knocked on our door and entered Nancy's hospital room. Cedric and Erin introduced themselves. They were from the hematology lab, the one that handles bone marrow transplants. Cedric was carefully carrying a small IV bag in his arms like it was a newborn baby. Erin had a black, large briefcase-sized shoulder bag containing equipment. Cedric immediately stepped up to Nancy's bedside so that she could see what he was cradling with his left hand while protecting it with his right arm.

The contents of the bag were bright, glow-in-the-dark red, like the AraC chemotherapy medicine. Since Cedric was holding the bag close to his body, its intense scarlet brilliance made quite a contrast with the long, white lab coat he was wearing. Jayna, Nancy's sister, Linda, and I had anxiously been waiting since early in the day. Erin quickly read the inquisitive look on our faces and explained, "We didn't receive the donor specimen until 6:30 p.m. tonight. I'm sorry it took us so long to get here."

I looked at the clock. It was well past midnight. Jaret was already back in his dorm asleep because he had two classes in the morning. October 27, rather than the originally expected October 26, would now be the "date of record" for Nancy's new beginning because of the lateness of the hour.

"Is that all I get?" Nancy inquired, sitting forward in her bed and leaning to her left for a closer look at the small bag in Cedric's comforting embrace.

"Yep," Cedric replied, shuffling his feet. "But let me explain what's happened so far. When the specimen reached us, there was over a liter and a half of fresh bone marrow material. It was collected early this morning and flown here from somewhere in the United States, probably back east, but we're not sure. We've been processing the bone marrow ever since it arrived at the lab. First, we drained off the fat and bone products. Then we put it in our spinner. Next, we siphoned off the stem cells that form at the top and ran tests for infections like hepatitis. Finally, we separated as many red blood cells from the stem cells as possible. We are left with mostly the stem cells that are right here."

Cedric's face beamed as he looked proudly at the bag he held close to his chest. He rubbed it gently, as if it was a baby's head.

"Well, just how much is in that little bag? It's pretty tiny compared to any of the IVs I've been given the last nine days."

Before Cedric could answer, Erin chimed in, "Almost two ounces. Fifty-three ccs to be exact."

Less than two ounces?

In my hand was a standard Pepsi can, twelve ounces. That's six times more fluid than the IV bag that was in Cedric's hands. I couldn't help but think how could such a tiny amount of fluid be worth the ordeal of the last five months?

"Are there enough stem cells to help Nancy?" I blurted without thinking.

"Absolutely," Erin announced, highlighting each syllable loudly. "Each cc in this bag contains about 340 million stem cells. Nancy will get more than enough to give her a fresh start."

When Erin paused, Cedric added, "Approximately 8 cc of the 53 cc are red cells we weren't able to separate away without damaging the stem cells. They cause the very bright-red color. And those red cells will probably cause a minor reaction because Nancy's red blood cell type is different from the donor's. But 8 cc is an acceptable amount, so Nancy's discomfort shouldn't be too great. All she should feel are a few aches and chills."

Erin finished her paperwork and double-checked the numbers on Nancy's ID bracelet. She handed the transplant bag to our nurse, Chris, using both hands so there was no chance the bag could be dropped inadvertently. Chris willingly accepted the offering with two hands, added the IV tubing she had prefilled with normal saline solution, and hooked the tubing into Nancy's central line, the special IV that enters her right upper chest and drains directly into a large vein below her clavicle.

"Well, Nancy, are you ready?" Chris asked as she looked at the wall clock (now almost four hours ago) and recorded the time, 12:37 a.m., on the form that had been placed on Nancy's night table. Chris had a smile from ear to ear—just like Cedric and Erin.

A bone marrow transplant, while not a major surgical operation like a kidney or heart transplant, is still dramatic. The science behind this potentially life-altering moment spans literally decades. And the logistics in our case of finding an unmatched donor and getting the "little red bag" to Room 507 at the University of Utah Hospital in Salt Lake City had been formidable.

Everyone in the room heard Nancy's audible gulp.

What could she be thinking? I thought silently. I squeezed her slightly sweaty hand between both of mine. Her resolute blue eyes looked squarely into my eyes. She didn't even have to ask.

Yes, I was ready even though my hands were now moist like Nancy's. My mind raced almost out of control and I silently thought to myself:

What if our donor had been hit by a truck on the way to the hospital?

What if the plane carrying his sample had crashed unexpectedly?

What if, of all days, an earthquake struck the Wasatch Fault today?

A multitude of unpleasant and usually catastrophic possibilities dominated every moment I wasn't engaged in direct conversation with Nancy or the others in the room. Each thought gave me pause. And through them all, I attempted to appear normal.

Once again, I thought silently—*Is this what schizophrenic voices were like?*

Erin finally broke the silence, "Did you know that to get your one and a half liters of bone marrow, your donor endured more than 150 sticks?" She pointed to her left hip. "Right here."

Despite all my research, I hadn't uncovered that particular detail. I would have been even more frantic had I known what the donor endured for my Nancy. Such worries, though, were now officially over. The red miracle fluid was being hung on its own IV pole as Erin spoke. The tiny life-giving cells were alive in our plastic bag. A crash to the floor couldn't jeopardize Nancy's chance for a cure.

Chris turned the dial to begin the flow of bone marrow after handing the tubing to Linda, Jayna, and me so it would pass through each of our hands before going into Nancy's chest. The 53 cc of mostly stem cells slowly dripped from the IV bag. The red stem cell fluid mixed with the clear liquid in the tubing and trickled down toward Nancy, lying in bed with her head elevated on three comfortable down pillows. I said a silent thank you to our "angel" donor as I watched the stem cells pass through first Jayna's, then Linda's, and finally my hands. In seconds, the leading red edge of the fluid entered Nancy's body. The entire tubing was now red, stem cells marching dutifully through her central line.

"Please find a suitable home," I prayed silently.

"Do you feel anything, Mom?" Jayna asked softly.

Nancy looked at Erin and Cedric and then each of us. "Relief," she answered, imparting the cheerfulness we all needed.

Jayna and Linda had moist eyes. Though my contacts did their job, Nancy wasn't wearing her lens. A tear ran down her left cheek.

"Mommer, don't cry. You're getting a brand new immune system. I know you'll make it."

"What makes you think that?" Nancy inquired, getting her own tissue. None of the rest of us dared remove our hands from the tubing.

"Because you're so strong. Look how you've made it through chemotherapy." Linda definitely agreed. Her shoulders appeared ten pounds lighter.

"And so nice," our nurse Chris added. "I've never had a patient thank me when I give her a shot."

Nancy frowned slightly so that her eyebrows pointed downward and her forehead wrinkled: "But I'm soooo old. Even though today is my new birthday." We all laughed. (According to bone marrow tradition, from this day forward, Nancy will consider today her "other" birthday, the day her new bone marrow was born.) No longer frowning, her face was glowing and without tears.

Emily Post doesn't have a chapter on how to act at a bone marrow transplant party. We sang "Happy Birthday Baby, Baby" several times and small parts of any other song that more than two of us knew. Jayna even made a video of our second rendition of the transplant shuffle, though Nancy danced with her arms only from her bed, the rest of her body beginning to ache. We made toasts (with water), and everyone but Nancy ate the chocolate "birthday" cake that I brought for the occasion, as well as the candy and cookies Jayna had picked up at the store.

By the time our neighbor's nurse stuck his head in our room and good-naturedly threatened, "I've already given my patient two 'sleepers.' Can you tone it down just a bit?" we were all emotionally spent and ready to settle down. Chris returned to other duties, and Linda and Jayna kissed Nancy good night and departed to our Sugar House (Salt Lake City) apartment.

When our room was empty and it was just Nancy and me, we did something we had not done since May 29, the day of Nancy's diagnosis. We discussed the future. We talked about what we will do once Nancy is well. We talked about trips that we'll take together. We talked about restaurants we'll visit. And most importantly, all the people we'll thank from the bottom our hearts—each and every one of you.

Summary: Last night, just after midnight, Nancy received her new bone marrow. We had a very special party to celebrate her transplant "birthday." If all goes well, we look forward to many, many more.

All our love,

Winnie

The One Redeeming
Quality of a Crocodile

November 13, 5:13 p.m.

Dear Friends and Family,

When I went to work yesterday, my longtime medical practice partner Chris Hays handed me a hatbox wrapped in Charlie Brown's Snoopy wrapping paper and a frilly blue bow. Over the past several weeks, I've been spending day and night in the hospital except when in the office, and I don't readily know one day from the next. Everything is a blur. So I quickly checked my "mental" calendar.

No, it wasn't Christmas.

No, it wasn't my birthday.

It wasn't even something obscure like "Doctor's Day." It was simply an act of kindness. Predictably, I was speechless and could barely get my thank you out without accompanying tears.

There were two pairs of new shoes inside the box, one for me and one for Nancy—Crocs. If you're not familiar with them, they are basically rubber clogs. Chris told me they are the "rage" and that they're everywhere. He went on to explain that Crocs are available in seventeen different colors. For me, Chris chose sage green. To my eye, they were more like the color of garden peas. (Unfortunately, I hated peas growing up. And I still do.)

Crocs look a little like Swiss cheese except for the soles. So, my new shoes are pea green and full of holes. They are definitely not a fashion statement. On the positive side, Crocs have one extraordinary redeeming quality: they "feel" really good. The holes allow your feet to breathe. And the rubber bottoms? Those flexible, spongy soles make them exceptionally comfortable. For that reason, my pea-green, hole-filled new shoes now reside in Nancy's hospital room closet. I haven't given Nancy hers yet, as she declared a moratorium on presents last week because she doesn't have the strength to respond with what she calls a "proper" thank you. But she really likes mine and was quick to observe, "Chris is a really close friend. He knows your favorite color."

Summary: We continue to be showered with love and kindness. Yesterday, Chris Hays gave me some Crocs. I have needed a new pair of shoes and will wear them comfortably as I stand ever vigilant and watchful over Nancy.

Warmly,

Winnie

The Angels Were with Us Last Night

November 13, 7:00 p.m.

Dear Friends and Family,

Earlier, I abruptly stopped writing my last letter because Nancy's "awake" times are now measured in minutes not hours. A little while ago, Nancy was awake only for about twenty minutes—normal for her over the last week or so. She has had a difficult time as a result of the chemotherapy she received before the transplant. The past week or so has been really challenging. And last night was one of those nights.

"Winnie, I need to go again."

Over the past two hours, Nancy had made numerous trips to the bathroom. (Actually, about every fifteen minutes.) It's a side effect of her medicines. She is taking three separate types of drugs to combat germs.

Antibiotics.

Antivirals.

Antifungals.

Each drug trickles into her body from a separate IV bag. Nancy is not allowed (nor does she want) to eat or drink anything. I find myself wondering if the medicines are the culprits causing havoc. I ask myself, "How can she have such a voluminous output when she feels the way she does each day?" Though, by 2 a.m., I stopped worrying about the causes. All that matters is helping her make it through the night.

"Winnie, it's time again."

I slip Nancy's feet into her fur-lined slippers and offer her my elbow for stability. I slide her IV pole carefully to the bathroom door while protecting the three IV lines that connect from the pole to the IV site in her too-thin chest. After situating her in the bathroom, I close the door and pace outside.

When the time that has passed seems longer than usual, I open the door. I can't believe my eyes. Nancy is there, but she's kneeling on the floor next to the toilet—cleaning.

"Sweetheart, you can't do that. You have no immunity. The germs could harm you."

"I'm only trying to get the worst of it."

"Stop! Please, let me do it."

Nancy doesn't argue. She's totally exhausted, but she is still thinking of others.

Quickly, I hurry into the bathroom to grab her before she collapses on to the floor.

After Nancy's next two "visits," I play housekeeper once Nancy has been returned to her hospital bed. And I do discover another great thing about my Crocs. They are easily cleaned in a sink with soap and warm water. They dry fast, too. (Chris, I find myself liking the color more with each passing hour.)

Our nurse, Erlene, finds me on my hands and knees cleaning the bathroom floor as she enters our room for the third time, bearing Nancy's nighttime medicines. After hearing my report, her eyebrows nearly hit the ceiling: "Oh my, Nancy. We do appreciate you wanting to help, dear. But cleaning the bathroom is not your job. It's ours."

My sigh is audible and I welcome the news wholeheartedly. Nancy doesn't argue with Erlene like she does with me. Erlene carefully places the drugs she is carrying on top of the medicine cart. She points at Nancy, and then me: "You are the patient, Nancy. Your job is to get better. And Winnie, you are the caretaker. You are not responsible for washing and scrubbing the bathroom floors."

"Well," I think to myself and almost say out loud, "I'm glad that's now clear. I might have forgotten who has the leukemia and who the caretaker is." Nancy scans the room for a place to go into hiding, but not finding one, nervously giggles. Erlene and I join her.

"Good you can still laugh, dear," Erlene adds, while hanging the next "bag in a long line of IV bags" that will be replaced tonight. "I bet you already know this, Winnie. Your wife is amazing. Everyone who's taken care of her loves her."

Surprising news?

No.

Almost every hospital worker who has assisted and helped us over the past five months has told me Nancy is his or her favorite patient—of all time.

"My dear, dear Nancy. We all want you to get well, but you can't risk that bathroom germs could get in the way of your recovery." Erlene turns on one of the small lights above Nancy's bed. It is one of the six different lights surrounding Nancy that allow her to have a "little" or "a lot" of light. "You look achy tonight, dear. Let me get you an extra dose of pain medicine. It's also time for your nausea medicine. Would you like that, too?"

For the next twenty minutes, Nancy's snoring filled the room and then she woke up for her next bathroom visit. Afterward, while tucking her back into bed and kissing her head lightly, she opened her eyes wide. (It's almost as if Brad Pitt, her favorite movie actor, had just walked into our room.) She grabs my hand and points in the direction of the door, "You have to give them a tip, Winnie."

"I don't know that the caregivers are allowed to accept tips, Nancy."

Not that each and every one of our nurses doesn't deserve something.

Uniformly, our nurses have been spectacular.

Uniformly, our nurses have been caring.

Uniformly, our nurses have been attentive.

Uniformly, our nurses have been knowledgeable.

And like tonight, uniformly helpful.

Erlene was stern this evening. Yet she has a playful and a kind touch. She turned a tense situation into a moment of amusement. She obviously understands how hard it is for Nancy to know that her body has changed, to have parts not work, and to lose her privacy. In reality, Erlene does deserve a tip.

"Please, Winnie. Please give her a tip right now—before she and the others leave. I hear them out in the hall."

As I search my briefcase for my wallet, I notice Nancy's head bobbing up and down. I stare at my bride in disbelief and then realize Nancy is dancing to music that only she can hear. I don't hear a single note.

"Nancy, I think Erlene and the rest of the nurses aren't in the hall right now. They are somewhere else helping other patients."

Nancy wrinkles her forehead and shrugs her shoulders: "Don't be silly, Winnie. You can't tip nurses. I mean the lady who put on the magic show."

"The magic show?"

"Yes. It was my favorite part of the entire performance—the last act of the circus. Right over there by the window." Nancy points to the window and I hear a childlike laugh that warms my heart. "Didn't you see it, Winnie?"

A circus?

"I missed it, sweetheart."

"Darling, what I think you saw was something like a dream."

"I think what you saw, Sweetie, was caused by your medicines."

"Honey, I think what you saw was caused by the extra pain medicine and the nausea medicine that were given to you at the same time."

Nancy replied matter-of-factly, "Oh, am I hallucinating like that other time?"

As Nancy rubbed her beautiful bald head, she added, "Whatever, I'm really sorry you didn't see the little boys and girls dressed as angels. They were the best. They were flying around the room. You didn't see them?"

I simply smiled and kissed her head again.

It was a long night, but despite Nancy's discomfort, despite feeling totally vulnerable, despite the fevers, despite the nausea, and despite the pain, Nancy (with all her inner strength) still finds ways to joke and have a little joy. And later Nancy vividly described the evening to Jayna and one of our favorite nurses, Colleen: "Their costumes sparkled, Jayna. Green, blue, and red sequins glimmered in the three spotlights coming from different sides of the room. You know, I'm still not sure the angels weren't real."

And while I'm not sure either, many of you have mentioned sending angels to watch over us.

Surely, the angels were with us tonight.

Summary: We are in a difficult period where Nancy's body is struggling. Still her spirit is strong—as is your continued support. I am eternally thankful for both.

Fondly,

Winnie

Nancy Has Begun Drinking Again

November 17, 10:37 p.m.

Dear Friends and Family,

"Dad, great news."

Jayna is at the hospital and I am, unfortunately, at work. It's just shy of noon, the time typically that Nancy's medical team makes their daily rounds.

"Dr. Peterson was just here. He thinks Mom is really improving. He said she could have ice chips and water—up to 500 cc per day, which is a little less than a can and a half of soda. She is *sooo* excited to be able to drink something!"

"That's fantastic!" I all but shout into the phone as if Jayna can't hear me. Nancy has been continuously thirsty this past week. She has constantly been denied water because her gastrointestinal system has been so fragile. Her lips have multiple painful cracks even though we have been applying emollient almost constantly. "I can't even imagine going an hour without drinking, let alone a week."

"And guess what else, Dadder? Mom's making white cells again. Finn Bo says it's the beginning of Mommer's engraftment."

It may surprise you, but sometimes I'm too emotional to speak. So quite honestly, I said nothing in response to Jayna's wonderful news. However, amazingly Jayna didn't miss a beat.

"It's OK, Dadder. We'll talk more when you get here tonight. And we'll celebrate—all three of us. We'll have a water toast."

Part of my toast will be for all your support. Thanks.

P.S. I may not have mentioned it recently, but Nancy has not read any of my letters. She does know that I try to keep our extended family and her many supporters informed, and occasionally she urges, *"Please don't include that in whatever you're writing about me."* Mostly, she ignores me while I wait for her to open her eyes or when I awaken in the middle of the night. All she occasionally sees is that I am busy on my computer. (I can only hope that if any of my writings are too graphic or too personal, you'll set my letters aside quickly and permanently.)

Summary: Nancy is finally coming out the other side. This week Nancy hit rock bottom, but she now appears to be on the upswing. Nancy is making new white cells. (Something that the doctors call engraftment is beginning.) She will soon be armed with new immunity and her new A-positive blood type. We are also expectantly awaiting her gastrointestinal tract to function properly again. With each passing day, Nancy feels stronger and better.

With much love,

Winnie

The Two Unspoken Words

November 20, 11:45 p.m.

Dear Friends and Family,

I'm frequently asked, *"Why are you working?"*
The answer is simple.

My days at the office continue to be a source of great personal satisfaction and, on some level, an escape for me. My partners, along with the rest of our amazing staff, sincerely care about Nancy. Many of them have known her for more than a decade. They also deeply care about me. Each and every day, they gently offer encouragement and support. They have learned not to ask me too much because they have learned that I write more easily about Nancy's and my situation than talk about it. They treat me normally except for the fact that they have assured me that it is all right if I have to leave suddenly or not come in to the office at all.

But then, there are my patients.

In a small town, word spreads quickly and pervasively. An incredible number of my patients now seem more intent on showering me with love than on having their medical complaints examined. Each day they bring me food. Each day they bring me presents. And almost every day they tell me their stories about loved ones who have also had a serious disease and survived.

When I take a moment to reflect on all those around me, I realize that every good thing I have ever done in my life has come back to me tenfold. The decent and noble side of humanity humbles me. As a doctor, it makes it all the more meaningful to me now when I can help others. The only trouble I have every now and then is when a patient inquires about Nancy. It is not uncommon for my bottled up emotions to spill out uncontrollably. Often it is one of my patients who is handing me the box of Kleenex or putting a hand on my shoulder rather than the other way around.

I don't mean to say that some days are not challenging.

Sometimes the rollaway cot in our hospital room doesn't provide me with the best night's sleep and I am physically tired when I get to the clinic office. Similarly, I feel the same way on those days when I have to take my shower at the clinic because the one at the hospital is being cleaned or fixed at the time I would normally use it. And then there are those days when I arrive at work only to discover that I have forgotten to bring clean socks or a suitably matching shirt. In reality, living at the hospital half time is not the best match with my job. But all things being equal, my greatest difficulty is when my mind and heart are still at the hospital even though my body is at the office.

Today was a day when I really wasn't at the clinic.

Why?

I never truly know. Sometimes I think perhaps it's because I'm at the end of a difficult period. As an example, today was my fourth consecutive day working. I found that I was instinctively calling the hospital every few hours.

"Things are fine, Daddy. Mommer is sleeping. She feels at least as good as yesterday, probably a little better. The doctors even advanced her diet. She's now allowed to drink up to 500 cc, and she can finally have something besides plain water. She just had her first sip of 7-Up. She smiled and said it was like sipping champagne."

After work, during my late-afternoon ride to the valley, I didn't ring Jayna, as is my habit. I felt like I had pestered her enough with my calling almost hourly. Instead I called Nancy's brother, sister, mother, my sister, and two of Nancy's best friends. (I have retrofitted our Subaru with a Bluetooth speaker so I can keep both of my hands on the wheel.) My daily drive to the hospital, thirty-five minutes from my Park City office or an hour from Woodland, is the best time to keep in touch. Everyone appreciates the news—especially today.

"I'm on my way to the hospital from work for an overnight with my bride," I tell them. "Jayna's been there all day. She says Nancy's a little better. Nancy's had three days in a row of good progress. Her new immune system is beginning to work."

When I stroll through the door, I announce my normal greeting, "Hello, my sweet girls. How's everyone doing?" I gesture and immediately wave a sign of my love to Nancy before turning to Jayna, who is sitting on the bed by the window. Instantly, I am frozen in my tracks. Jayna is hunched forward and she is sobbing uncontrollably.

The next ten seconds last an hour. Blood rushes to my face and moisture slickens my hands. My head starts to pound and my legs struggle to keep me upright. I begin to get angry. It can't be. It can't be.

How could Nancy's leukemia return?

A single tear is balanced on Nancy's cheek as I race to Nancy's bed and grab her exposed hand, but there is no horror on her face, unlike mine. Nancy is mouthing a word. I bring my ear closer in an effort to enable her to whisper a single word: "Alain."

After I delicately place a quick kiss on Nancy's beautiful bald head, I move to the other side of the room. Alain is Jayna's Peruvian boyfriend. I attempt to comfort her by stroking her thick hair and by holding Jayna's trembling body close to me. In a matter of moments, I can feel dampness from her tears on my shirt.

"His visa was denied, Dad. What are we going to do?"

As you may remember from earlier letters, Jayna was in Peru when Nancy was diagnosed with leukemia. Jayna had just completed her junior year abroad from Vassar, the college in New York that also sponsored her "year abroad" program. When I called, Jayna responded immediately by returning home the very next day. She's been at her mother's side ever since.

Most of you know that Deer Valley Resort is one of the three local ski areas on the east side of the Wasatch Mountains. My very good friends at the resort had kindly arranged a winter job for Alain. So today, with a work offer in hand, he was getting ready to leave his family for six months in Utah.

We later discovered he had traveled 350 miles by bus from his home in Cusco, Peru, to the American consulate in Lima, but the US bureaucrat in charge of his final paperwork wouldn't authorize his entry into the country.

I must admit, even though Jayna was hurting as I held her and stroked her hair, I was momentarily buoyed and completely thrilled. Then, just as quick, I became a basket case of conflicting emotions. Initially, all I could think of were the two words that every cancer patient most fears—*"It's back."*

At the outset, all I saw in Jayna's puckered brow and disconsolate sobbing was a brush with disaster.

Why?

How could I feel relief that Alain is sitting in Lima?

In the end, I realized today that Nancy is my everything, but so are Jayna, Jaret, and everyone else in our extended family. Ultimately, we formulated an alternate plan. I called my friends at Deer Valley Resort and they jumped into action. They made several phone calls to their Peruvian contacts and Alain is now scheduled for a second interview and chance—which is all any of us can ask.

At long last, Nancy is lying in bed with a new immune system and no sign of recurrence. Three weeks have passed since her transplant. She's had no serious infections. And most importantly, the two words everyone in our family fears, *"It's back,"* have not been spoken.

I can make you this promise: we'll be ready for whatever next week brings.

Summary: When Jayna's Peruvian boyfriend was denied passage to this country today, I was reminded that Nancy's disease also has had major effects on the other members of our family. I will redouble my efforts to support Jayna and Jaret.

My very best,

Winnie

The Engraftment Blues

November 22, 9:13 p.m.

Dear Friends and Family,

Each and every day, we wait expectantly.

I almost never go to the cafeteria, even if my stomach growls, murmurs, or gurgles. I won't go even when I crave a chocolate croissant. If I visit the bathroom at the far end of the hall, I always run both ways. I never want to miss the best time to ask questions and, sometimes, to hear answers from the doctors as they make their daily "rounds," the time our medical team comes to see Nancy.

What did the urine culture grow?

How is Nancy's liver holding up?

Can she eat a piece of toast yet?

Should her medicine dosage be changed?

Every facet of Nancy's care is discussed during the rounds. (It seems so strange being on the opposite side of the bed. I've been part of a similar team my entire career.)

On rounds yesterday, our new attending physician, Dr. Pulsipher, pulled an index card from his back pocket. Smiling, he proclaimed, "Nancy's platelet count this morning is up to 107,000. We can d/c (discontinue) her platelet transfusions. She's now making her own." He pauses, looks for confirmation from Jayna and me, and gives Nancy a thumb's up: "This is the first concrete sign of engraftment."

Isn't it funny how a single number can change your entire outlook?

My whole body was suddenly warm and I fought back what seems at times to be my never-ending battle with tears. (How

231

can I still be so emotional after nearly six months?) The reality is that I know too much. Though far less than 1% in bone marrow transplant patients, if engraftment fails, it is gravely serious. In both fact and reality, it means "game over."

"And Nancy's absolute neutrophil count is 420," Dr. Pulsipher continued. "That means she is beginning to produce white cells, too."

The role that platelets play in our bodies is to stop bleeding. Nancy has received them regularly the last two weeks because she had none of her own. But white cells? There is no such thing as a white cell transfusion. White cells fight infection. The "black cloud" of a deadly germ attack has hung ominously in our room for the last two weeks. Evidence that Nancy is now making her own infection-fighting cells is, in a word, *huge*.

"Once your white cell count is above 500, you've regained the ability to fight infections. And when you stay above 1,000, we can start taking away your IV antibiotics."

I really fought my emotions at this point, and I bit my lower lip as my contacts suddenly got too blurry for me to see Nancy's face.

"But when will I feel better, Dr. Pulsipher?"

Sometimes I forget that Nancy assesses things differently from me. (Numbers to her are only mildly interesting.) She may (or may not) ask me to explain a lab value like, "What's a BUN?" She may (or may not) even reflect on what I have said even after I tell her: "Oh, now I understand. A normal BUN means my kidneys still function like they're supposed to work" However, what makes Nancy happy is far more basic.

"When will it stop hurting to roll over?"

"When will my stomach accept food?"

"When will I feel better?"

Despite today's lab numbers that made her medical team proud, Nancy is still struggling. She is still achy, nauseated, and tired.

"And why do I feel worse if my numbers are so good?"

"You have to realize, Nancy, there is an awful lot going on inside your body. As you produce white cells and immunity factors, your body may feel worse because your tissues are healing. We've blasted you with very powerful drugs to kill your leukemia. But the drugs are also very toxic. It will take a while to recover. We even have a special name, the 'engraftment blues,' for what you're experiencing now. The engraftment blues are the time period when we are happy with how things are going and when we see your transplant starting to work. But it's also when you don't feel as good as you will soon."

"The engraftment blues?"

I saw in Nancy's face that she really understood.

"Fine," she said.

"Can we do anything more for you today, Nancy? How about if we adjust your night meds so you can sleep better?"

"I'd really appreciate that, Dr. Pulsipher."

The team doubled Nancy's pain meds. So last night Nancy actually slept better than I did as I tossed and turned on the rollaway. She slept right through the shrill alarm that sounds every time there is air in her IV line or when one of her many medicines finishes. Her eyes remained closed when the nurses came in and out. Not even soft kisses on her head stirred her.

On today's rounds, Dr. Pulsipher congratulated Nancy again: "You are officially engrafted, Nancy. Let me be the first to applaud your progress. Your absolute neutrophil (white blood cell) count is 1,740."

"That's great. Last night I slept the best I have in a long time."

"I'm so glad to hear that. Now it's time to start eating. If you want to leave the hospital, your absolute neutrophil count must be above a minimum 500 for three days in a row—which shouldn't be a problem given today's numbers. You can't have a fever or sign of infection, and you must be taking most of your nutrition by mouth. It's time to start working on that last requirement."

"What can I eat?"

"We'll start off slowly. Today you can have mashed potatoes or rice. If you can, try to eat at least one slice of toast. And no more restriction on the amount of your clear liquids."

Nancy and I had two water toasts tonight before bed.

Our first salute was to a landmark day—Nancy's engraftment day.

And our second tribute was to all of you.

P.S. In all honesty, we made a third toast to Sarah Ann Ezzel, a childhood friend of Nancy's from Georgia. Sarah Anne visited Utah this week and provided some incredible help filling in for Jayna at the hospital. Nancy reveled in reliving memories from her past. (A pleasant escape from the present?)

Summary: Today was a very important day, Nancy's engraftment day. According to her blood tests, her transplanted donor stem cells have finally set up "residence" in her body. She is now producing the cells she needs to move forward. Now we're anxiously waiting for her to feel as good as her improving daily lab numbers.

Thanks for everything,

Winnie

One More Bite of Oatmeal

November 26, 7:47 p.m.

Dear Friends and Family,

When our attending, Dr. Pulsipher, arrived for his rounds today, he stunned us: "What would you think about going home on Wednesday? You can have a real Thanksgiving."

Jayna and I looked at each other and I have no doubt that we immediately shared the same thoughts.

Are you serious?

That's only forty-eight hours from now.

She still sleeps night and day.

She just started eating yesterday.

She couldn't even take a single sip of water three weeks ago. (And when she did take a sip, she had a better than 50/50 chance of having the water come back up!)

Are you just trying to get her home before the holiday?

Nancy responded first, "Do you think I'm really ready, Dr. Pulsipher? I'm still a little tired."

"If things keep going like they are, you'll be fine. Just keep up your eating."

"I'm trying, but it's really hard. I don't have much of an appetite even though I'm less nauseated almost every day."

"That's normal. Think of it this way—a Mack truck has run over your intestines. That's the effect of pre-transplant medicines. You're actually doing great. It'll just take a little while longer."

After the doctor left, I found myself wondering again about how long "a while" is, but my beloved partner answered the question by lunch. Nancy simply devoured everything on her plate—like every other challenge. Today she chose a new primary focus—food. And her target was oatmeal.

"I want to eat the whole bowl, Winnie. Can you add more sugar?"

Nancy's words were somewhat mumbled, and I was only able to decipher her question because I was sitting close to her. I pieced together her desire only by piecing together her individual words and the situation. Her eyelids were open only enough to reveal the enticing blue underneath them. Though I added two sugars as fast as I could tear the packets, Nancy was snoring by the time the frosty white coating covered the remaining cereal.

"Sweetheart, do you want more?" I asked softly as I put my hand on her shoulder.

Nancy struggled to reopen her eyes; it was almost as if glue was preventing her from opening them again.

"Did I doze off, Winnie? I want to finish."

I fed Nancy six more bites, reminding her to open her mouth and chew after each bite because she fell asleep after each one. As she looked down at a finally empty bowl, both of her shoulders rose for a deeply breathed sigh. Determination. An instant later, Nancy was back in dreamland.

She is going to be discharged in less than three days?

For her next meal, Nancy ate mashed sweet potatoes. But this time, it was without my help. "I'm practicing for Thanksgiving, Winnie. These potatoes actually taste pretty good."

Chemotherapy has made everything taste different for Nancy. When I ask, Nancy summarizes her experience in this way.

"Most things taste bad."

"The grape juice tastes like metal."

"A bagel feels like cardboard when I swallow."

To Nancy, it doesn't matter because leaving the hospital is her goal. Her first bite most often causes a reflex frown, but then every swallow is followed by a triumphant smile.

Summary: Nancy has embraced a new goal—eating enough to be released to our Salt Lake City apartment in time for Thanksgiving.

Love,

Winnie

A Real Reason to Give Thanks

November 29, 6:50 p.m.

Dear Friends and Family,

By yesterday, Nancy could eat a full portion of something three times a day. She can now eat a banana, a cake donut with chocolate glaze, or some orange sherbet. There hasn't been any vomiting or any diarrhea for more than four days. Most importantly, her IV food and fluids had nearly been discontinued.

"Are we really leaving the hospital today, Winnie? I'm a little nervous. I can't imagine not being in bed, looking out the window at our lovely view of the mountains."

I think to myself and admit silently, *"Neither can I, my love."*

In fact, I can't imagine taking Nancy to our new apartment. At this point, Room 507 feels secure, and I now take for granted that Nancy has made a significant transition. The blinds in Room 507 are always open now. Nancy is focusing on things outside our room. She's come such a long way

Suddenly, I flash on a comment Nancy made at one "loopy" overmedicated point when she sat up abruptly from a deep sleep and declared, "I love this hotel room, don't you?"

As I marvel at the view outside our window with Nancy, I also look at our many personal decorations. I must admit that I, too, have become attached to Room 507. Even though I have to walk the long hallway to reach the bathroom several times a day and even though it represents our scariest phase to date, Room 507 really has been a decent home.

In spite of this sentimentality, it's time for us to take the next step. Nancy is willing. Once again, I am the one who is least prepared. My mind races like a stock car at the Daytona Speedway.

What will we cook?

How will we measure Nancy's oxygen level and blood pressure?

What about her temperature readings?

Do we even own a thermometer?

"I can't imagine it either, Nancy. I've gotten pretty good at being a nurse's assistant's assistant. I've even learned how to make hospital corners on your bed."

In our apartment, Jayna and I will assume all nursing duties. But I face an even bigger worry and bigger questions.

Will I be forced to serve as Nancy's doctor?

What if I have to decide if something is trivial or serious?

Why is this so much harder—it's our fourth exit from the hospital since Memorial Day?

"Time to get the bins, Winnie. If we're leaving, I want to be out before the clock strikes midnight. Let's get packing."

I turn toward the origination of the laughter and look into Nancy's eyes—finding them especially bright. She knows. I kiss her head and she squeezes my hand with both of hers. I speak to her with just my eyes, as only a couple that have been married for as long as we have can. My moment of doubt is over, Nancy. I'm eager to blow this place, too. Let's hope it's the last time.

With my newfound energy, I decide to jog to the car to get the bins. As I stand up from my chair, the medical team enters the room.

"Hi, Nancy, did you have a good night?"

"How are you feeling?"

"Much nausea?"

"Any diarrhea?"

"How tired are you compared to yesterday?"

I hear these routine questions but notice that the oncology fellow and the pharmacy resident standing behind our attending, Dr. Pulsipher, are shuffling their feet. They avoid eye contact.

Dr. Pulsipher finishes his questions, acknowledges Jayna and me with a nod, and then states, "Nancy, your liver enzymes took a jump today. We don't know why. We're thinking maybe we should postpone your departure until we sort this out."

Nancy makes an audible sigh before quickly gathering herself and responding, "Oh? Really? What do you think's happening, Dr. Pulsipher?"

"I suspect the rise is a reaction to one of the new oral medicines. But we want to be sure it's not graft-versus-host disease. We should be able to tell in the next few days. We can shoot to get you out of here by the weekend. Can you make it to Saturday?"

Nancy's look of disappointment quickly blends into a sunny smile. "Uh, I guess so. Sure."

How does she do it?

My stomach instantly contains a knot.

Disappointment?

No. Much more.

Worry.

"Dr. Pulsipher, how likely is the enzyme elevation graft-versus-host?"

"Well, Winnie, Nancy has a 70–80% chance of developing graft-versus-host at some point during her recovery. If the graft attacks her liver, you will see the enzymes go up. More often, you see an elevation of her bilirubin level, and she will get jaundiced and turn yellow. That's not happened. So right now, I'd have to say GVH (graft-versus-host) is not very likely. But we don't want you to leave the hospital and have to come right back."

"I agree. That would be devastating." (I don't say more devastating, though, truth be known, that is how this news has left me.) "Thanks, we'll adjust. There's nothing like Thanksgiving in the hospital."

"Actually, tomorrow you should plan on a pass. Leave for a few hours and have a nonhospital meal. The more Nancy eats the better."

"Don't worry, Dr. Pulsipher. I'm sure I'll eat a lot tomorrow. I even liked the taste of something the other day. What was it, Winnie?"

"Sweet potatoes."

"Well, Nancy," Dr. Pulsipher responded with a smile, "Plan on lots of sweet potatoes. I'll be in to see you early in the morning so you can leave here at a decent hour."

I endure another long night as I constantly find myself thinking about Nancy's elevated liver enzymes. I wonder if the lab finding is trivial or the beginning of significant liver damage? I rationalize that Nancy has done so well, better than anyone anticipated. Her meds certainly could be the culprit. Almost every one of them is processed through her liver. But what if it's graft-versus-host disease?

Much to my delight, Nancy awakens when the early morning rays touch her face. (Remember, we haven't closed the blinds in days.) Recently, she's slept through sun, all the room lights, and most of the noises that emanate from the hallway outside our room. Nancy barely says good morning before she confirms today's plans: "Winnie, guess what? I actually feel hungry. I might try some ham today. Happy Thanksgiving!"

"Perfect! Jayna is already at the apartment cooking a ham for you. I can't wait. Happy Thanksgiving, sweetheart."

Dr. Pulsipher and the fellow from oncology interrupt our conversation before Nancy and I have an opportunity to talk about the rest of our day ahead. Not surprising, given the holiday, they are without their normal entourage of students, nurses, and other medical professionals. Even better, they are a full hour earlier than their usual time for visiting Nancy.

"Good morning, Nancy and Winnie. We've decided against you going out on a pass. We want to discharge you instead. Your liver enzymes are nearly normal this morning. The elevation must have been a transient reaction to one of your new medicines. Congratulations!"

November 29, Thanksgiving.

It is a day that will forever be remembered in the Winn family archives. Our family will not only be together, but we will be together outside of a hospital. We will breathe nonfiltered outside air and feel direct, unfiltered natural sunlight. Within an hour, Nancy is riding in our car beside me. She has remembered to fasten her seat belt and she is listening to the radio, just like a normal person.

At the apartment, there is no need for a tray to be placed on Nancy's lap. She is sitting at a real dining room table. Her bed is actually in its own separate room. No more bells or buzzers. No interruptions. No IV pole.

Freedom.

Nancy eats her home-cooked ham on real dishes. She adds salt to the sweet potatoes from a saltshaker that is not disposable. Her silverware will go into a dishwasher rather than a trash basket. She asks for seconds on sweet potatoes that are served from a dish on the table.

Thanksgiving.

After just under a month and a half confined to a single hospital room, our holiday meal together is as notable and enjoyable as the step through the revolving hospital door that we playfully went around in twice as we were leaving today.

Still I can't help but wonder if everything will be "normal" now?

It is too early to know.

But there is one thing we know for sure: we know that we have many things to be thankful for.

P.S. Alain, Jayna's Peruvian boyfriend, was denied entry to the United States for the second time. We are unable to figure out why. Jayna has had quite a year, but she too has much to be thankful for.

Summary: Happy Thanksgiving to each of you. Believe it or not, we are no longer in the hospital. We enjoyed a fitting holiday celebration after forty-three days in the hospital. Nancy is thirty-three days post-transplant and still has no serious infection and no significant organ damage. She does have a functioning, brand-new immune system. So today I "froze" a snapshot of our family with the camera that is my memory. Today was a Thanksgiving that none of us will ever forget. We have much to be thankful for—Nancy's present health and our deep and abiding friendships with each of you.

Fondly,

Winnie

A Jumbo Pillbox

December 4, 1:06 a.m.

Dear Friends and Family,

At times, the last six months have played like a horror movie or, at the very least, a recurring bad dream. Each and every day, we have faced relentless fears that are continuously lurking in the shadows. Our emotional highs and lows switch places then are swapped again and again. Our unrealistic hopes are frequently vanquished by the harsh reality of Nancy's disease. We have lived day to day, hour to hour, and sometimes even second to second.

As a result, we analyze and reanalyze every word uttered by our medical team. We worry each time Nancy has her blood drawn. We hold our breath when Nancy's temperature is taken, and we don't sleep when she has the cancer-checking bone marrow biopsies done. Each day contains its own drama, so we savor even a few hours of blissful sleep as an escape from what is an almost surreal existence.

But this week, with being far away from the constant reminder of residing in the hospital?

I must be honest.

Our days have been resplendently dull.

On most days I wonder, how can a patient with arthritis do it?

I wonder, how does someone that is a touch forgetful get through the day?

How about a person with poor vision?

The answer to all these questions—the pillbox.

On the day we were discharged recently, I made the compulsory trip to the hospital pharmacy. Since it was midmorning on Thanksgiving Day, I had the entire place to myself. I should have known what would happen.

"Oh, so you're Nancy Winn's husband. I've been expecting you. Her order's been ready since yesterday. We were so busy we didn't have one spare moment to breathe. We spent a considerable amount of time getting your order ready and then you didn't come."

Yes, my hair was disheveled as usual. And no, I hadn't showered or changed clothes since spending the night on my chair in Nancy's hospital room, where I had fallen asleep before I could get up and go to the rollaway bed. The "look" the short, round-faced, redheaded pharmacist gave me above her thick reading glasses made me want to hide. Her face was dripping not with turkey gravy—but with disdain.

"It's not our fault," I wanted to say. "I would've been here yesterday, all cleaned up and on time, but our discharge was postponed—by our doctor, not me. I was devastated and worried yesterday, so I didn't clean up today because I want to get out of here before our doctor changes his mind again."

I knew whatever I said would fall on deaf ears. So I settled for, "Yep. That's me. I go by Winnie. Do you have my wife's pills for us?"

The pharmacist rolled her eyes in concert with a slow shake of her head. She straightened her nametag, which read in bold, black letters "Cynthia."

What I really wanted to say was, "I know, Cynthia. I know, it's Thanksgiving Day and you're working. But have a sense of humor. It's Thanksgiving and we've been in the hospital for almost a month and a half. Can you just take a deep breath?"

"These are your wife's medicines—the entire bag. And it's heavy." She plopped it on the counter with a large thud to make her point.

She was right. The bag was filled right to the top. Some of the items in it were quite large, like the box containing Lidocaine numbing patches for Nancy's persistent sciatic back pain. Mostly, however, the bag contained pill bottles of varying sizes. There were lots and lots of them.

It was a good thing the pharmacy was empty. The next twenty-five minutes were spent discussing side effects. Cynthia never looked up once and she barely took a breath between holding each pill container up near my face as she read from her many sheets in her never-ending monotone. After the last one, she shoved the bag and a piece of paper across the counter: "Sign here."

After a "thank you" that was not acknowledged, I grabbed the bag and cradled it like a football under my left (dominant and stronger) arm. Somewhat unsettled by my pharmacy experience, I didn't mark the significance of my final exit through the hospital's revolving door like I did when Nancy and I went around twice before I took her to the apartment and then returned for the drugs. No wonder. My head was spinning like the door. How will Nancy take all these medicines? (As I shared with you previously, she gets queasy from a single sip of water.)

When I arrived back at the new apartment, we had a long and warm four-person family hug with Jayna and Jaret, who had been busy preparing dinner. Jayna looked at her mother lying on the couch and said, "Go to sleep in your bed, Mommer. That one is mine."

Jaret added, "I'm setting the table, Mom. You and Dad both look tired."

He was right. So I tucked a weary but happy Nancy into her own nonhospital, queen-size bed. The down pillows that cradled Nancy's head showcased nonwhite pillowcases (two blue and one pink). The bed was a simple luxury even if it didn't adjust into eighteen unique positions like those in the hospital.

I kissed Nancy's shiny head and then gently stroked her bald dome until her eyes closed and there was a steady rise and fall of her chest. In contrast to the blue and pink pillowcases, the hairless part of Nancy's head was almost as white as her teeth. It was a beautiful contrast, one that I had not noticed surrounded by the hospital room's white pillows, white blankets, and white walls during the last month and a half. I thought to myself, "How nice to have color back in our lives." And then I whispered, "What color will your hair grow out to be this time, Nancy?" Nancy didn't answer.

With my first task accomplished, I celebrated by quietly pulling a chair up next to the bed and propping my feet up next to Nancy's. It suddenly occurred to me, "How delicious to do nothing but watch Nancy sleep."

It's just too easy to adjust to no interruptions.

Or cleaning floors.

Or taking vital signs.

Or inventorying equipment.

Or giving Nancy her meds.

Meds, I thought with a jolt?

The brown bag I had placed in the corner when I arrived at the apartment earlier looked back at a face that was just about overwhelmed. Reality set in quickly and I opened the nightstand drawer and pulled out the recently purchased, four-times-per-day, "largest-in-the-Western-world" pillbox. This particular organizer is capable of holding a full week's worth of medicines. I slipped out of the bedroom and sat on the couch, arranging all the pill bottles to the left of the pillbox on the coffee table in front of me. No doubt we needed the Super Walmart of pillboxes. The coffee table barely had room for the water glass Jayna brought me. As she set the tumbler down, she raised her eyebrows and commented, "It looks like I have the easy job today, Dadder."

The next sixty-eight minutes were occupied putting nineteen different medicines into slots representing the four time periods Nancy is supposed to take her pills each day.

Morning.

Lunchtime.

Dinnertime.

Bedtime.

When I made my final count, thirty-three pills per day had found a home in Nancy's weekly pillbox. Thirty-three. There have been entire years when I haven't taken thirty-three pills. From the tiny blue one that will probably land on the floor more often than not to the capsule that is just a tad smaller than a hot dog, I carefully deposited each pill into its designated space. With each pill in its labeled time slot, I rechecked each niche a second time. Not surprising, I discovered I had made four mistakes.

A rustling of blankets emanated from the bedroom. After a moment of silence, a sleepy-sounding voice could be heard: "Winnie, is it time for me to take a pill?"

For the foreseeable future, there is an easy answer to Nancy's question.

"Yes, sweetheart. I'll bring you the entire pillbox."

Summary: Nancy is single-handedly keeping the pharmaceutical industry afloat financially. Luckily, we found the world's largest pillbox to organize a full week's worth of her medicines at a time.

All the best,

Winnie

Ask and You Will Get Answers

December 5, 5:51 a.m.

Dear Friends and Family,

I had a long phone conversation the other day with our dear friend Patricia. She asks many of the same questions that many of you do, so I thought I'd repeat some of my answers for today's update.

"How's she doing?"

"It's remarkable to be discharged thirty-three days after an unrelated donor transplant, even for a younger patient. She's come such a long way and been through so much. Nancy has had four separate extended hospitalizations. But now, she's getting a little better each day."

"Will she need to go back a fifth time?"

"We don't know—that's why we're required to live close to the hospital in Salt Lake City. Each week, we return to the hospital several times. Fortunately, we only go to the outpatient clinic. We hope never to be admitted to the hospital again. We hope no problems come up during this phase of Nancy's recovery."

"Any problems?"

"Yes. Though we're out of the hospital, there are still challenges. Nancy has her donor's immunity now. But by design, it's being suppressed to ease it into her body. It's like being able to only drive a new car under sixty-five miles per hour for the first 1,000 miles. You might call it the 'break-in' period. So with Nancy's new immunity not yet at full strength, infection is still a major concern. It's nowhere near the way it was before the transplant when she had zero immunity, but Nancy still needs several medicines to protect her against germs. She even has to wear a mask if she goes outside the apartment, which makes it hard to go to a restaurant or movie.

"During the next two months, the immunosuppressing medicines she is taking will gradually be withdrawn. As that happens, Nancy's other major risk comes into play. It's called graft-versus-host disease, or GVH. While the donor white blood cells were a 10/10 match with Nancy's, they are still designed to attack things that are foreign. Everything in Nancy's body is foreign to her new white blood cells. Once she is off immunosuppressants, the donor cells might attack her skin, bowel, liver, or other organs."

"When will you know if she has that graft-versus-host thing?"

"Nancy is thirty-nine days post-transplant. By day one hundred, we should have a pretty good idea. We've been told to expect some graft-versus-host disease, but we hope for a minor amount. Seventy to eighty percent of patients Nancy's age gets some graft-versus-host.

"Finally, even though Nancy has survived four long hospitalizations for maximal chemotherapy and the bone marrow transplant, there is always the chance that her leukemia will return. It will be a couple of years before we can feel safe that she is cancer free.

"All that said, Nancy is making steady progress. She is able to eat more at each meal. She is increasing her exercise one minute every few days. She is waiting for her body to heal, so each week there might be fewer pills in the world's largest pillbox."

P.S. For those who have asked for our Salt Lake particulars: Nancy Winn, Apartment 3, Sugarhouse Village Inn Apartments, 1339 East 2100 South, Salt Lake City, Utah, 84105. I still travel to Woodland at least once a week for the mail, to water the plants, and to pick up clothing that Nancy now wants to wear. We have a phone in our apartment, but we haven't bothered to even find out the phone number. However, our mobile phones do work in the apartment. Nancy actually does answer her phone on occasion, but even when she doesn't, she always smiles when she listens to your messages.

Summary: Psychologists list "moving" as one of life's major stresses. The relocation to our apartment in Salt Lake City has been just the opposite. Nancy's enjoyed a quiet, peaceful period since leaving the hospital. She is "homing in" and getting used to being normal. Each day, I see increased well-being—both physically and mentally.

With much love,

Winnie

The Merry-Go-Round Goes Round

December 11, 8:50 a.m.

Dear Friends and Family,

I realize my letters have recently been less frequent; when Nancy came home to her "real" home, I didn't expect to write you for weeks. I had hoped to spend all my nonwork time assisting Nancy in her recovery. Quite honestly, I thought most of what was happening in our corner of the world would be blissfully boring. Mostly, my plan was to sink my teeth into transforming the Salt Lake City apartment into a proper "second" home.

To me, it's more than a bit amusing how I now view time and space. In the past, I would never have entertained transforming a hospital room into "home." Or that I'd even consider making a "temporary" apartment into a place for celebrating the holidays and life in general. Simply, I was used to one place to hang my hat and call my home. During all the years I spent summers in Yellowstone, I never once hung a picture on the wall. I'm almost embarrassed to admit that sometimes I never even unpacked my suitcase to use the chest of drawers.

But now?

I am so much more anchored to the present. Or at best, the very near future. Even as a doctor, I never quite realized it. Cancer (or any other serious disease) totally changes your perspective. Cancer forces you to be flexible. Yesterday is a great example of what I am trying to share with you—just when I had scheduled to spend a full day of being at home, events conspired to alter my plans. When I walked in to the house, Nancy was on the phone about a more important matter. She wasn't making calls about holiday decorations and preparations.

"Nancy, we probably should have you run up to the hospital for a few tests. Yes, right now. Do you want me to talk to Winnie?"

"There's no need, Adam. That's why we rented the apartment in Salt Lake City—to be close."

Nancy had been feeling increasingly tired the past two days, and her temperature has been rising today. I was happy to hear that someone besides me would be checking her—and since it was Adam, the nurse practitioner on call for bone marrow transplant patients, she would at least bypass the emergency room.

(For those of you who don't know, transplant patients go straight to the bone marrow outpatient clinic conveniently located on the hospital's fifth floor. The clinic is only a few steps away from the specialized bone marrow transplant hospital rooms, just in case.)

"Winnie, I'm fine. I want you and Jaret to go to Woodland as planned. Jayna can take me to the hospital. Jaret's looking forward to being at the house and my plants need watering. Besides, I need some warm clothes for going outside. I want that sweater with the Santa Claus on it. You can always come back down if this is more than a minor problem."

In Nancy's typical style, she put her plants and Jaret before any concerns of her own. An hour after our Woodland arrival, she did the same thing again.

"My fever is higher than we thought, Winnie. So Adam wants me to stay in the hospital a few days. He said my 'army needs a few weapons' it doesn't yet have."

I paused for a long moment and Nancy immediately responded, "Winnie, Winnie. Please don't get all emotional on me. I'm not planning to die yet." Right on cue, I heard her almost childlike giggle, which made it nearly impossible not to smile.

"Jayna's here with me and says she'll stay tonight. Enjoy your time with Jaret. You can sleep in the hospital with me tomorrow. It will be just like old times. In the meantime, find all the clothes on the list I gave you before you left the apartment. And I would like the treadmill back up here at your earliest convenience."

Nancy's muted sense of humor made me smile again. The "treadmill" has become part of the Winn family legend. When

Jayna first had the bright idea to buy a treadmill for Nancy's room after her transplant, Nancy protested, "I will never use it." Those were strong words from Nancy; she was dead set against it. But we thought that it would be beneficial, and with Jayna's help, her mother's stance softened. A week later, the hospital staff marveled when a hospital engineer inspected and put an "official" sticker on the fold-up NordicTrack C2200 treadmill that had just been delivered to our room. We placed it neatly in the far left corner facing the window to take advantage of the spectacular view of the mountains.

As I signed the purchase papers that day in the hospital room, the delivery crew told me, "Oh, by the way, this is a first. We've never made a delivery to a hospital patient. There is no delivery charge—this one is on us. We hope your wife is better soon."

Jayna and I used the treadmill every day after that and a week later, when Jayna and I returned from a brief cafeteria run, we found Nancy gingerly walking on it. "Don't either of you say anything," she stridently cautioned Jayna and me. "What a view!"

So given her less-than-positive response to our original gift, I felt unencumbered and unrestricted in my response, "Well, Nancy, I guess if you want the treadmill there, you can't be too sick. I guess if Jayna promises to call . . ."

"Jayna, will you call Dad if I get worse? Winnie, she's giving you a thumbs-up. Now go watch a football game with Jaret and then get some sleep."

After saying good night, I hung up without responding further to Nancy. "That's easier said than done," I verbalized to what was now a disconnected phone. With my feelings unbridled, I grabbed two Kleenex boxes for my nightstand. Though the football game was an agreeable distraction, the rest of the night was filled more by questions than answers.

Should I have noticed something sooner?

Did I bring home a bug from the office?

Have I kissed that beautiful bald head too many times?

When I finally dozed off, sleep was not friendly. Germs that looked like termites from a Terminix TV commercial marched through my dreams. The new apartment was full of them. They covered the walls. They covered the floors. They marched in a straight line from behind the couch toward Nancy, who was lying in bed reading a book. When she turned a page, they jumped on her from between the pages and were joined by their brothers-in-arms who were ascending the bed. Time and time again, she attempted to swat them away but could only look at me with a frightened and terrified face.

In another dream, I lay next to Nancy in bed, but somehow I was running on the treadmill. Before I could come to Nancy's rescue, a giant germ jumped in front of me, poised to bite. He had four protruding eyes and twenty or so hairy arms and was fully a foot taller than me when he stood on his hind legs and made a hissing sound. He was so horrific; I awoke with a jolt. I sat straight up in bed, palms and forehead sweaty, trying to get my bearings in the middle of the night.

I didn't attempt a return to my dreamland because being awake was easier and less stressful than being asleep. Instead, I ventured out on the deck to watch the sun peek its brightening orange head above the eastern horizon. The early morning light revealed a thick gray mist rising from the frozen river. It floated eerily upward into the snow-covered branches of the nearby trees and, given my recent dream, was more chilling than I would have liked under different circumstances. After all, Woodland was normally my safe place.

As the sun's rays increased in intensity, they created sparkling reflections in the snow. In every direction outside the bedroom windows. I witnessed nature's beauty, which lifted my spirits. Two deer, a mother and daughter, casually walked by to drink from the part of the river that wasn't completely covered with ice. The morning magic embraced me, wiping away the night's bad memories. The giant germ was just a distant recollection, and after much consideration, I decided not to bring the treadmill back to the hospital.

Summary: I have been "off the grid" because it has been a calm time. No longer. Last night Nancy reentered the hospital with a fever. I will write later when I know more. Thanks in advance for an extra positive thought about Nancy today.

Much Love,

Winnie

Balancing on a Tightrope

December 11, 6:02 p.m.

Dear Friends and Family,

It was a welcome sight to see a friendly familiar face when I arrived on the fifth floor at the University of Utah Hospital today.

"Good to see you again, Winnie." Lisa, like the other nurses and personnel on the floor, still remembers us. Though it seemed like a long time ago, it's only been two weeks since our last hospital stay.

"Does she still have a fever, Lisa?"

Lisa looked at the floor and said somewhat hesitantly, "39.7, Winnie. Bless her heart."

"Guess you're still providing the heat in here, sweetheart," I told Nancy as I entered her room and kissed my favorite, now somewhat disarrayed and fuzzy head.

Even without a fever, Nancy warms any room. But 39.7 degrees Centigrade? I quickly did the math in my head. 103.5 degrees Fahrenheit. In an infant, that is a very high temperature. And when I discuss a 103.5-degree fever with the mother of one of my pediatric patients, I usually say, "It feels like I could fry an egg on your daughter's stomach."

But Nancy?

My wife, as you well know, is not in the pediatric age range—103.5 degrees is very high. During my medical training, a fellow resident contracted measles and had a temperature similar to Nancy's. His fever caused a seizure and he hallucinated.

So Nancy's fever, in and of itself, is scary—but even scarier are the three critical questions such a temperature raises:

1. Where is the infection?

2. Is the infection viral or bacterial?

3. And most important, will it respond to treatment?

Jayna has learned more medicine in a few months than many students do in their first year of medical school. She was quick to report that the required tests had been completed. She also assured me that Nancy's IV contained "big gun" antibiotics.

With luck, Nancy's fever is merely the signature of an everyday virus.

With luck, Nancy's fever will leave her as quickly and mysteriously as it arrived.

With luck, Nancy's fever will depart, leaving Nancy unscathed.

Immediately, I thanked Jayna for the information and gave her a hug. I also did the best I could under the circumstances to pretend that I was not having "bad" thoughts, because I was (once again) in the distasteful position of knowing that I know too much.

So why would I be so concerned?

Nancy's immunity is barely forty-five days old. If you imagine her immune system as a brick wall, the bricks are there, but the mortar is still lacking. There is a specific part of her immunity, the T-cells, that not only needs to grow and mature, it will need to not be suppressed by her medicines as it is now. The balance between infection and graft-versus-host disease is a daily tightrope that now may be unbalanced.

Currently, Nancy remains in good spirits, continuing to make me laugh during the brief periods she stays awake. Though very weak, she is quick to reassure me that she has no new or significant pain. A few moments ago, she laughed ever so lightly and said, "I can't wait to get back on that treadmill."

Summary: Though we are back in the hospital, Nancy's spirit is strong and she is not in pain. We are anxiously trying to determine the cause of her fever while hoping that it will respond to treatment.

Love,

Winnie

So You Think You Can Dance?

December 18, 6:41 a.m.

Dear Friends and Family,

Our hope for a "short stay" in the hospital has faded like a winter sunset. Each ray of distant hope has been replaced by a cold reality.

Simply, we're still here in the hospital.

Even though it is wonderful that Nancy is not receiving any "poison" chemotherapy drugs as she has in the last three hospital stays, this hospitalization has two very undesirable similarities to her initial trip to the hospital.

First, this visit was not scheduled like her other chemotherapy stays. It is entirely open ended. Regrettably, we have no idea of how long she will be in the hospital.

Second, during the other times Nancy was hospitalized, the focus was the treatment plan and hoping there were no major side effects. Now, like her first hospital admission, the focus is discovering the reason for Nancy's symptoms and then, if possible, treating the root cause.

Consequently, this round seems considerably more ominous and it is very difficult for me to keep my chin up. But with Nancy to buoy my feelings and the great medical care we continue to receive, I hope to soon report that we are on our way home.

A story that began last night best illustrates our situation.

"Is your dance card full, my lady?" I say to Nancy after she alerts me she is in need of my help.

My comment elicits more than a smile from Nancy. After feigning a search of our mostly darkened room, Nancy bursts into a long, full laugh. (I still marvel at her amazing spirit. If you touched me, in contrast, I would break into a thousand pieces.)

"No one else here, Winnie. So I guess you're stuck with me."

As I wrap Nancy in my arms, I can't help but feel the intense warmth of her 102.8-degree fever. I slowly guide her small, uncertain, shuffling feet until we reach the bathroom door as I cherish our closeness. I think to myself what a great idea. She's not unsteady when I hold her like a dance partner. (Her previous trip to the bathroom was nearly a disaster. When she stumbled, I barely caught her in time to prevent what could have been a catastrophic fall.)

On the way back from the bathroom, I elicit a second laugh from Nancy with my off-key rendition of *Strangers in the Night*. We reached her bedside still in the dance position.

"Let's do that again, Winnie. Probably within the hour."

Nancy places a full kiss directly on my lips. Not a small kiss, mind you. Not a peck on my cheek. The room almost spins in the semidarkness. I feel like I've been transported back to the senior prom. "You must really be delirious, Nancy."

It's been a long time, my love.

"I'm not delirious. It's my way of showing you how I feel."

"You feel hot. You need to get back beneath the covers. You're shivering."

By the time I stretch four heavy, white blankets underneath her left arm and right foot, Nancy is asleep. I place multiple soft kisses on that beautiful bald head, barely visible in the light from the IV pump.

"Winnie, can I have another dance?"

I can't help but think to myself as I get groggily up in the dark of our room, *Already, Nancy? It's three in the morning and it's only been twenty minutes.* Then more awake and with my wits more fully about me I say, "Let me help with your slippers, sweetie."

"Hurry . . ."

By morning, my exhaustion is overshadowed by deeper and darker emotions:

Apprehension.

Melancholy.

Fear.

Sunlight from the east heralds day seven of this hospitalization. It already is more than double our anticipated three-day return to the fifth floor of the University of Utah Hospital. Nancy has endured repeated blood tests, cultures of every part of her body, and multiple X-ray scans in search of a germ and where it might be hiding. So far, each examination has been negative. Good news, yes. However, each test is a search for an unwanted culprit.

Uncertainty extracts a large toll psychologically on both the caregiver and the patient. Nancy's forehead wrinkles are now more visible. Her uplifting giggles are less frequent. She doesn't want to be alone for long.

"What do you think this means, Winnie? I truly enjoyed our dances last night, despite your singing. But a bathroom waltz every half hour? Do you think my diarrhea will ever slow down?"

As I begin to formulate answers to Nancy's tough questions, Richard enters our room. The most flamboyant of our nurses, Richard is usually more like our maître d' than one of the hospital staff. Today he waves both hands in a full circle like a prop plane's propellers as he glides gracefully toward Nancy.

"Hello there, Winns," he says as he snatches up each of the four different juice boxes on Nancy's bedside table. Then with a police officer-like voice, he declares, "Nancy, you are officially NPO (nothing per oral). No more fluids or food for you. You have graft-versus-host disease in your bowel. We have to rest it beginning immediately."

Nancy's mouth drops and tears form in both eyes, which no longer sparkle.

As an uncontrollable wave of heat races through my body and my face flushes I blurt out, "What are you saying, Richard?"

"Winnie, what I'm saying is that Nancy's bathroom problems are indicative of GVH disease. Almost every allotransplant patient gets GVH—especially if they're older than forty-five. The likelihood is something like 80%. Don't look so shocked. Graft-versus-host disease isn't all that bad. A little GVH protects against a leukemia recurrence."

I want to immediately ask two questions: "How do we know Nancy's GVH will be a 'little?'" and "Why does it have to be now?" But I don't ask either of my potential inquiries as I look at Nancy's face and see that she is devastated because she has had her heart set on celebrating Christmas away from the hospital. My questions are not asked because I don't want Nancy to hear the answers, and I realize that I'm not sure if I want to know the answers either. I simply hold Nancy's head to my chest.

Richard saunters from the room with Nancy's drinks, nodding his head since both hands are filled.

"I'm thirsty, Winnie." Nancy murmurs. "I was just starting to taste things again."

For a moment I feel like I'm watching a Mideast peace report on TV and everything is hopeless. I even fantasize about tackling Richard before he closes our door and pilfering at least one of the near-empty drinks from his hands. Instead, I say, "It's all right, Nancy. GVH is just a new minor detour. You're flexible, right?"

"I guess I still have leukemia, don't I?"

Minutes later, our attending physician, Dr. Pulsipher, entered the room and confirmed our new concern: "We need to be sure about what's happening to Nancy's GI system, Winnie. We probably should do a colonoscopy as soon as we can reverse her blood thinners. If at all possible, we'll shoot for tomorrow. I've already talked with Dr. Herbst, a gastroenterologist who works with our patients, and asked him to biopsy Nancy's bowel. The pathologists can look at the tissue to see if immune cells are attacking it and then we can be sure about the diagnosis."

"And if it's GVH?" I whisper so as not to awaken Nancy.

"We will begin treatment. GVH is graded from one to four, with one being mild. If it's mild GVH, we will simply rest her gut. If the grade is above one, we will start steroids."

I sank very low in my chair as I heard this not welcome news.

"Remember, we expected Nancy to have GVH sometime and somewhere. Today is day fifty-two post-transplant. Again, let me remind you that it would be very common for her to have it."

The next night, Nancy slept better than I did and we had far fewer "dances." The good news is that her temperature remained normal for the entire night. So I left for work in the morning and headed to the mountains tired but encouraged and cautiously optimistic. Then several hours later, between seeing patients, I received a different update when I checked in with Jayna.

"Well, Dadder, Mom is feeling bad again. Her fever is back. The doctors are still worried about GVH. They want to study the upper part of her bowel on Monday if things don't turn around."

It has been a week of ups and downs. And this morning, Nancy expressed her disappointment and sadness. She described doubts and demons that constantly lurk in the back of her mind. Yet, like always, she recovered with new resolve and her incredible capacity to think of others.

"Winnie, now that I've gotten that off my chest, you know what I'm thinking? Everyone should be enjoying Christmas, not worrying about me. Maybe you, Jayna, and Jaret should go to Woodland for Christmas. What do you think?"

What do I think?

I think I have an incredible partner. I think that today I will try not to worry. I will just enjoy her company. And I think we will laugh at the thought of spending time away from Nancy during the holidays.

Summary: Nancy's fever slowly disappeared early this week. We have no answers as to why the fever came or what caused it. With no evidence of infection, our path took a different turn. Our new worry is graft-versus-host (GVH) disease. A colon biopsy was another dead end, but Nancy's symptoms continue and her fever is back.

With concern,

Winnie

The Best Christmas Ever

December 20, 8:38 p.m.

Dear Friends and Family,

As a medical doctor married to an airline flight attendant, our family has over the years often celebrated holidays at nontraditional times and in nontraditional places. Every year since the kids stopped looking up the chimney for Santa Claus on Christmas morning, I have volunteered to work on Christmas Day to allow my younger partners at the clinic to spend family time with their children. Many years Nancy was flying on Christmas, and other years she and the kids went to her mother's home in Georgia. So Christmas for us has always been a "variable" holiday. The only requirement became finding a time when Nancy, Jayna, Jaret, and I could be together in the week before or after this special day.

This year will be different.

The frozen image outside our surprisingly large window at the hospital could pass as a Christmas postcard, and the snow-covered mountains seem close enough to touch. A nearby residential development shows off homes twinkling and dressed in holiday decor. Beyond the homes and mountains, the sky is painted in red, orange, and gold as another day comes to a close. However, inside Room 506 at the University of Utah Hospital, it is anything but a normal Christmas. There are no live bowls of holly and no Christmas cookies. In fact, there is no food at all.

How are the holidays for the Winn Family?

Yesterday, I realized that we would not be leaving the hospital any time soon. "Dadder, don't be so worried," Jayna told me as she studied my face. "Think of it this way: The doctors have always said Mom will likely develop GVH at some point. Why not get it over with now? I don't want to go home and come right back. Do you? And besides, if we end up being here on Christmas Day, who cares? It will be really easy for Mom. Can't you just imagine her at the apartment, fretting over not having enough presents for Jaret and wondering if the shirt she bought you is a color that you'll actual like—let alone wear? If we stay in the hospital, we can do all the work. Mom can just stay in bed and enjoy things. Cheer up. Chill and take a look at the tree Emmy brought us today. It's so cute. Christmas in the hospital won't be so bad."

I couldn't help but think, "My dear, sweet Jayna. You're grown up now and you lift my spirits in the same way your mother does each day." With some real effort required on my part I responded, "The tree is cute, Jayna. It's not even three feet high. And it's a little different from the ones that touched our ceiling when you were still leaving notes for Santa."

During our children's early years, we would annually venture into the forest to cut a tree with the Fields, our neighbors. Many of our holiday trees stood over twenty feet, and decorating them took two ladders and sometimes a full week to get the lights and ornaments just right. However, it was always worth it. Jayna and Jaret's wide eyes consumed their faces as they would race down the steps on Christmas morning.

"Mom really likes the small tree. When she woke up from sleeping and discovered it, she clapped her hands. We can do it, Dadder. This will be the best Christmas ever—even if the doctors do decide Mom has GVH."

Once again, I decided that it was best to keep my thoughts private. But I couldn't help but think silently: *All right, Jayna. We'll have a Christmas to remember, even if it's in the hospital. Where do I hang my fears? There's no tree big enough. Your mother looks so serene, asleep in her bed—but she's facing the two most terrifying challenges (infection or GVH) of transplant patients. Jayna, quite honestly, I don't know which diagnosis to wish for in my prayers. You think we should treat GVH now and get it over with, Jayna. Prednisone, a steroid Mom would take in gargantuan doses if her symptoms prove* to be GVH, is lifesaving—but prednisone is an awful drug. It affects sleep and causes temporary diabetes—and high blood pressure, skin changes, and weight gain. Yes, it would keep the new bone marrow from attacking Mom's gut, but the cost is very high. And most scary, a high dose of prednisone increases the already elevated risk for infection.

"You're right, Jayna. We do need an answer to Mom's fever and bowel problems—even if it's GVH. I just had hoped she wouldn't get it for a little while longer, preferably sometime after Christmas."

"Dadder, let's make plans then. What do you think we should get Mom?"

We can get Mom anything you want, Jayna. In fact, let's get her everything you and Jaret can think of for Christmas. Our holiday this year will never ever be surpassed. What's important is that we celebrate together, like always. This year Christmas should be one day that, unlike every day since this all began for Nancy, she'll truly want to remember always.

Summary: As Christmas approaches, it looks like Nancy will remain in the hospital. Her medical team is trying to figure out why she has fevers and a GI tract that won't accept food right now. Though disappointing, we will plan a big day in Room 506 and be very thankful that we won't gain any weight like we usually do during the holiday season.

Sincerely,

Winnie

Stepping Up Isn't Hard to Do

December 21, 10:36 p.m.

Dear Friends and Family,

Today after work I was ordered by my "girls" to go to Woodland rather than come to the hospital, as is my usual routine. "We want some girl time, Dadder," Jayna explained on the phone.

Nancy had a slightly different explanation: "Jaret's been alone for several days. He needs you more than I do. Isn't there a football game on TV tonight?"

Nancy was right; it was time for a trip to the mountains. Jaret met me at the door of the house, which is somewhat unusual for him.

"Hi, Dad. Did you have a hard day at work?"

"Pretty busy, Jaret. I'm sorry to be getting here later than expected."

"That's okay. The game doesn't start for twenty minutes."

"Who's playing?"

Over the last month, watching a football game with Jaret has become part of our Woodland "routine." We both anticipate and cherish the experience no matter what time I arrive home from work or the hospital. The teams don't really matter. The score doesn't matter either. What matters is the illusion of normalcy. After all, I'm usually snoring (loudly I'm told) by the second quarter. (I also come to Woodland more often these days since it is Christmas break at Westminster College and Jaret is home continuously for the next several weeks.)

"Dad, guess what?"

"What?"

"I already took out the trash and watered the plants. You didn't have to remind me. I even remembered the laundry that Emmy didn't do yesterday. And since you're working so hard, I did the dishes, too."

Jaret beamed and so did I. (With a normal child, news of this sort would be a pleasant surprise, but with Jaret and his unique challenges, such actions are major.)

"Thanks, Jaret."

"I want to do my part, Dad. How else can I help?" Jaret walked over and kissed my bald spot. (I can't help but wonder if it feels as good to Nancy when I kiss her head as Jaret's kiss did to me.)

"Jaret, you're already helping more than I could have imagined. Mom will be proud."

"Oh, I forgot to ask. How is Mom today? Did they find anything out?"

"Actually Jaret, I was just about to tell you some really good news. It's taken ten days, but they finally figured out what germ Mom has in her body. The biopsy of her colon shows CMV virus."

"Is CRV bad?"

"CMV, Jaret. Any infection Mom gets is potentially bad, but the doctors believe their medicine will kill the CMV virus. We'll see how everything works in the next couple of days. And guess what else? They also think the CMV virus is the cause of Mom's fevers. What that means is that if Mom has any GVH, it is mild. I really hope they're right."

Jaret was listening intently and his eyes were glassy like mine. Though he often has difficulty finding words, he has a deep love of his mother. He welcomed my hug with open arms. "Jaret, you need to know that Mom will be very excited to hear what you've been doing at the house. She'll be just as excited as we were when we learned about the CMV. Again, thanks for everything you do for your mother and me."

Summary: Even Jaret has stepped up in our struggle through these difficult times.

Excitedly yours,

Winnie

A Holiday Miracle

December 24, 11:09 p.m.

Dear Friends and Family,

Today we learned that even though Nancy is tolerating the medicine for CMV well and is slowly improving, it is now definite that Christmas Day will be spent in Room 506.

For the past few days, I have anticipated this news, but there is a part of me that had hoped for a Christmas miracle. However, we have quickly adjusted. On the twenty-fifth, I will (as usual) work, but my partners insist that I only work the second half of the day so our family can actually celebrate Christmas on Christmas Day morning. Kathleen, my partner, good friend, and riding companion, called me last week to inform me of my partners' decision. She said, "You've volunteered to work on Christmas Day for as long as any of us can remember, Winnie. This year, at least, you will come in late in the day. The partner group insists and won't hear anything different." Jaret, Jayna, and I have embraced this change and have immediately begun preparing for the big day. Even the hospital staff has noticed.

"Oh my gosh, Nancy. I don't think I've ever seen better decorations in a patient room."

Hope should know. She'd been a nurse on the bone marrow transplant floor since before Jayna was born over twenty-two years ago. A Christmas tree, Santa's sleigh, and a holly wreath that glitters in the afternoon sun are from my creative days when I made holiday presents out of stained glass and glass jewels. (Emmy, our Christmas angel, has provided almost all the other decorations.) Numerous strands of white lights camouflage the dull-brown hospital shelves. A basket of plastic branches and artificial flowers has turned the TV stand into a festive holiday display. Four bright Christmas stockings are hung from the towel rod behind Nancy's bed. Emmy told me they were her "extras." But I must admit, I wonder if it was a Christmas "fib." (Who in the world has four extra matching elegant Christmas stockings just lying around?)

Finally, there is our perfectly shaped "too-cute-to-be-true" little tree perched ever so preciously on Nancy's nightstand. It stands all of nearly three feet tall with short, stubby, symmetrical branches. Each branch drips with Emmy's miniature ornaments. (Where did she find miniature decorations?) The tree "matches" the holiday gift from Joannie, our neighbor and close friend, who cleans the cobwebs and everything else that needs it at our Woodland home once a week. Since Nancy will not be venturing outside, Joannie has sent a handmade miniature wooden snowman. Nancy named him "No Frost" and has found him a seat of prominence on the last available shelf.

A short while ago, Hope handed Nancy a present: "This gift was delivered this morning, and you are supposed to open it now."

Nancy read the handwritten tag: "We love you guys—our family is thinking of your family. Merry Christmas, Bob." Bob Evers is one of my two original partners. We built our medical practice together, even raised our families together. His children are the same ages as Jaret and Jayna, and both sets of kids shared many milestones and friendships.

When Nancy opened the present, she found a hand-carved ivory-billed woodpecker inside wrapped in tissue paper. One of Bob's many other talents is woodworking. The woodpecker's movable wings spanned over two feet and the highly polished body was made from inlaid maple and red heartwood. "It is so beautiful, Winnie. Can we hang it above my bed so I can see it all the time?" I stood up to fetch the fifth floor's ladder. "Wait," Nancy said before I could leave the room. "Listen to the note."

Nancy read slowly from a pink notecard with lacy fringe that she unknotted from around the woodpecker's neck. The card was written in calligraphy by Bob's lovely wife and

Nancy's very good friend, Anne. (You may recall that Anne is the lab tech who works at LDS Hospital, where Nancy was first admitted. She was the technician who took me to view the slides of Nancy's "bad guy" leukemia cells.)

The card read, "The ivory-billed woodpecker had last been seen in 1944. Hence, all of the major bird experts and bird books declared it extinct. Last year, however, it was rediscovered in a swamp in Arkansas. Birders called it a miracle. The bird is thriving today. Like the ivory-billed woodpecker, most thought you would be 'extinct.' Having this bird in your room symbolizes the miracle we expect for you." Each member of the Evers family had signed at the bottom of the note and sent their love.

Ten minutes later, our woodpecker was hanging from the light above Nancy's bed, adding to the Christmas spirit.

Summary: A hand-carved, wooden bird that vigilantly flies just above her hospital bed now protects Nancy. The ivory-billed woodpecker is our symbol of hope and miracles and also a reminder of the amazing support given to us by our friends and family.

Very much love,

Winnie

A Christmas to Remember

December 25, 9:17 p.m.

Dear Friends and Family,

First, and most importantly: Merry Christmas and Happy Hanukkah.

Our hospital room is deeply personal and extremely intimate today. It is not surprising that the fifth floor is quiet because every patient well enough to be discharged has been sent home for Christmas. Nancy is dressed for the occasion in her candy cane pajamas, Christmas socks, and no-longer-visible bald head. She is nonchalantly hiding it beneath a Santa hat, a present from her sister, Linda. (It's a way for us to be connected to Linda even though she is physically in Georgia.) Nancy's glowing face makes the room feel warm and fuzzy. Even though it's not the place we would have chosen for our Christmas gathering—we are off to a good start.

Jayna arrives a few minutes later, huge plastic bags slung over her shoulders. "Ho! Ho! Ho!" she utters in a deep and throaty voice as she drops one of the overflowing bags and spills the presents across the floor. Nancy and Jayna fill the room with laughter.

The ivory-colored phone on the portable stand besides Nancy's hospital bed rings. And rings again. And again. Uncharacteristically, Nancy answers the phone, and her eyes immediately tear up and become slightly glassy. The many voices she hears are loved ones from near and far away sending their best wishes. Every caller wants us to know they are thinking of Nancy and the Winn family. Nancy recaps each phone call to us, describing in considerable detail each person she speaks with and word-for-word their kind messages.

Jayna's two bags filled with presents double those already neatly stacked in the chair that guards the end of Nancy's bed. The chair is overflowing with offerings of varying sizes and shapes. I can't for the life of me think of who shopped, wrapped, and bestowed so many gifts for our family. The stockings are bursting with goodies that were also not brought by Jayna. Emmy must be the culprit. (She's not only an angel, she's a saint, too.)

The next hour or so is deliciously joy filled for the Winn family and, unlike any Christmas I can remember, it is totally relaxed. There is no table to set. There are no meals to prepare. Nancy sits up in her bed and Jaret, Jayna, and I take a seat along the edges of her blankets. During our "family" time together, we do not encounter any interruptions that would somehow disrupt the magic in our room. The hospital staff seems to know not to disturb us.

Nancy is somewhat hesitant to be the center of attention as we make "merry" in our little room. We snap picture after picture, making sure that anyone who sent Nancy a gift will see firsthand that she received it. We urge Nancy to model a new bracelet and hold up a new pajama top for the world to see. We toast to her new blood type by clinking water-filled glasses. And then I notice—Nancy's face looks like she has just received an injection.

"Shall we take a break, Sweetie?"

Nancy doesn't answer. Instead, her forehead lines soften as she rests her head on the pillow behind it and shuts her eyes. Initially, I fear that we have asked too much of Nancy and that we have worn her out with too much activity and commotion.

Ten minutes later, our nurse Hope tiptoes into the room, taking a somewhat circuitous route through all the wrapping paper, bows, and boxes haphazardly strewn on the floor. She taps Nancy on the shoulder: "I'm sorry to interrupt, dear, but it's time for your pills."

Nancy sits up and carefully swallows three white pills. She doesn't lie back down. She turns to Jaret, Jayna, and I bunched together on the one remaining empty chair and flashes a smile that nearly knocks me over. "Don't I have any more presents?"

You do indeed, my love.

She opens the final gift-wrapped packages, unable to alternate with us since we've long since opened the last of ours. In days gone past, Nancy was always Mother Santa. Inevitably, when it came to unwrapping gifts, Nancy was always the first one finished. But this is a very different year. It is time to write new Winn family traditions. Now we take more pictures, we talk of past holidays—and we share more kisses and hugs and water toasts.

"I got more than you did, Winnie. I also got more than Jayna and Jaret. How did that happen? It's not fair," Nancy declares when all the gifts have been opened and shown around the room by each "giftee."

"I remember a lady who once told me 'Life is rarely fair.' But as I recall, she wasn't bald back then."

I remove Nancy's Santa hat to kiss her head amid more merriment. The Santa hat is appropriate even though she didn't purchase a single present this year. Somewhat wistfully, I long to freeze the moment and the warmth I feel inside my body. All I can see is the happiness on faces that surround me. Unfortunately, moments in time don't freeze and the door opens unexpectedly.

"I guess it is a little late to say, 'Good Morning, Winns.'"

Julie Asch, our attending doctor, walks into our room with only two of the "regulars" from her entourage. The clock reads three-thirty in the afternoon. It is many hours past Julie's customary morning visit time. (Holidays in the hospital are different for the doctors, too.)

"I thought you forgot me today, Dr. Asch."

"Not a chance, Nancy. As you might imagine, I had some pressing family business this morning. I left a living room full of decorations and opened boxes to come see you." Dr. Asch gestures at our messy room. She is not wearing her traditional white coat, and she looks as relaxed as my bride. "Well, Nancy, I am 'Dr. Santa Claus' today. All your numbers look good, and your bowel seems to be behaving better. We can start full clear liquids this afternoon. And do you remember the winding tunnel I described to you yesterday—with twists and turns, and even an occasional dead end? I think we might be seeing the first rays of light at the far end. If all continues well, we may try to get you out of here soon—maybe sometime next week."

I don't believe that I've ever heard such beautiful words.

"Really?" Nancy's face brightens the entire room.

I bend over the bed, attempting to give Nancy's forehead a kiss, but she guides me to her lips. My legs wobble after so many weeks of being so cautious about spreading any germs to Nancy's weakened and compromised body. She whispers in my ear, "Winnie, this Christmas is the best ever."

As Jaret and I head for the door, I turn back and Nancy is already dancing with sugarplums. Her presents have disappeared from the bed, but the red Santa hat with white trim peeks out from under the edge of the green blanket. I think to myself as I walk to the car that, indeed, this is a Christmas to remember.

Summary: Today we celebrated Christmas inside the hospital. Unlike past years, we did not have a live tree, hot drinks were not served, and our traditional Christmas was not prepared by Nancy. But nonetheless, this year's holiday will be a Christmas we will never forget. Our family was together and joined in celebration as Nancy's condition improves.

With much love,

Winnie

Warts and All

December 30, 11:46 p.m.

Dear Friends and Family,

At long last, it's finally time to make a quick exit.

Since the current round of hospitalization had been unplanned, we didn't have much to load into the back of the Subaru, which made packing the car a snap today. Unlike previous "rounds" we hadn't brought any of the normal decorations. In fact, we didn't even have Nancy's pajamas to repack because when she was initially admitted, she hadn't planned on staying. And then, once there, we concluded, "Why bother?" (So we didn't! Everyone, including us, had hoped Nancy would be out in less than three days.)

We were really wrong this time, however.

This time, Nancy spent nineteen days in Room 506.

"How many times have we done this, Dadder?"

"Let's see." Even though the last seven months are somewhat a blur because I live mostly day to day, this particular statistic didn't require much thought: "This is our fifth hospitalization, Jayna. But only our second move back to the apartment from the hospital."

Going back to the apartment again was like watching the same movie for the second time. I noticed many things anew that had been missed upon my initial viewing. Coming back to the apartment was like seeing new characters, scenery, and dialogue. The steps from the car to the front door were longer than I remembered. (Especially after I made seven trips to bring in fresh groceries.) The front door didn't close easily and made a squeaky noise that will wake up everyone when I arrive

273

home late from work at the clinic. The kitchen appeared much older and smaller than when Nancy went back into the hospital three weeks ago. The purple-flowered wallpaper looked like something from the old TV show *The Adventures of Ozzie and Harriet*. (There isn't even an icemaker in the refrigerator.)

By far the worst aspect of the apartment is the room we have "designated" Jayna's bedroom. It's pretty obvious now, but we somehow missed its original purpose. Her "bedroom" was designed to be the dining room. It doesn't have any doors. And it can't even properly be considered to be part of an open floor plan because it is conveniently located in the middle of the passageway between the living room and the kitchen.

As I walked through Jayna's bedroom and put the last bag of groceries on the kitchen counter, I silently chuckled to myself about the many blemishes I now recognize in the harsh light of our return visit. With perspective, though, the apartment's character flaws pale in significance to what's truly important.

When I stop for a moment and glance into our bedroom, Nancy is already asleep. It is a deep and serene slumber aided by the realization that she is out of the hospital at last. I find myself smiling even though I know that the apartment will be our home for the next three to six months. In the future, no one will awaken Nancy to check her blood pressure. The only beep she might hear will come from my phone if I forget to make the switch to silent mode when I climb into bed late at night. She will be able to venture not only to a bathroom but also a kitchen, an ex–dining room/bedroom, and a living room with couches and chairs. She will be able to wear as little or as much clothing as her heart desires without the fear that a stranger will interrupt to check equipment or a medicine cart.

My reverie was interrupted when Jayna tapped me on the shoulder, grabbed my hand and lead me to the living room: "I know what you are thinking Dad. My bedroom is fine. We'll be fine."

Clearly our apartment has some now obvious warts, but at the same time, it also has some fantastic "smiles" that fill the apartment with happiness.

After all, in the end, what really matters?

Loved ones, family, and close friends are what matter in the world. We have made it through another crisis, and the love of my life, though weak and tired, is ready to resume her recovery.

I can say without any hesitation—I'll take the apartment every time, warts and all.

Summary: Though much of the luster is gone, we are pleased to be back into our Salt Lake City apartment and out of the hospital. We are upbeat at the moment and certainly hoping from here on out for a smoother ride.

Hopefully yours,

Winnie

Tonight's the Night

January 1, 1:17 a.m.

Dear Friends and Family,

Yesterday was day two in the apartment—December 31, the last calendar day of a very, very difficult year.

A large part of our day was spent watching Jayna modeling outfits for her mom. Finally, after what seemed to be hours to me, they agreed on a certain pair of jeans, new boots, and a light-blue sweater that highlighted Jayna's eyes and newly manicured off-blue fingernails. Shortly thereafter, Jayna gave each of us a kiss, saying "love you" as she raced out the door, leaving for a party scheduled from 2 p.m. until sometime into the wee hours of the night. Not surprising, Nancy had the satisfied look of a mother happy that her daughter was doing something normal for a twenty-one-year-old. In all honesty, I must admit I was equally thrilled as well. (And not to be forgotten, Jaret was already in Woodland, excited to watch his favorite shows on our TV, which is bigger than his.)

This year's New Year's Eve celebration was a bit different for Nancy and me. There weren't any specialty drinks (or even the slightest hint of alcohol), and there wasn't a sumptuous meal before midnight. (Nancy did tolerate two pieces of toast around noon. We even put a smidgen of butter on the second slice.)

Nancy did promise me a dance at midnight, though.

"Winnie, I want to see the ball descend in Times Square and hear 'Auld Lang Syne'—while we are dancing." When she made this request, I wondered if she knew that Robert Burns composed the song from a Scottish poem he had written in 1788 and that the title translates to "old times."

Nancy's promise to "dance the night away" was made a little over two hours ago, between taking her six bedtime pills and emptying the IV bag containing her nutritional supplement. She had expressed the idea just as I was completing the daily dressing change on her central IV line—the one that enters her body just below her left clavicle. Two days earlier, it had been a worrisome task because the site had looked red and ugly. Fortunately, the redness is almost gone now.

"Winnie," Nancy said as she grabbed my hand the minute the dressing change was complete, "I'm not forgetting our dance tonight, but I've been thinking. What would someone do if they had leukemia but were alone?"

"I don't know, Nancy. But you are definitely not alone. There's me, Jayna, and Jaret. And then there's your sister, and Emmy, and my sister Suzie, Janis, Mona, Julie, and Patricia. John, Fred, Anne and Bob. Sarah Anne, Joannie, June, and Marion. I could go on and on, my love. You've got so many helpers. There are scores of other friends just waiting for my call. I'm not even counting those far away, who have offered to help and are willing to travel to provide it."

"But some people are alone, and I could be. Don't you wish you were out having fun tonight?"

"I am having fun. It was a challenge tonight to get your dressing just right. And I couldn't be happier to see that the port site looks better now."

"Winnie, you know what I mean—the things normal people do on New Year's Eve. I wish you could do what you want."

"Nancy, Nancy—I am doing what I want."

As I kissed Nancy's beautiful bald head. I felt a prick on my lower lip. "What's this?" I asked as my index finger rubbed the new stubble that singularly stood straight up atop her head like a lone cactus in the middle of a too-dry desert. "Are you growing hair?"

Nancy's semi-frown transformed into a grin and she laughed out loud. Even after more than a quarter century of New Year's Eves, I felt true tenderness in the pit of my stomach and warmth in my heart.

"Seriously, Winnie. I hope you'll be able to enjoy things more next year."

"And I hope to have someone healthy to enjoy them with . . ."

"Do you know what my favorite New Year's was, Winnie? The year you, Jaret, Jayna, and I watched the Times Square ball drop during our early days in Woodland. We drank sparkling cider and Jaret was on my lap and Jayna was on yours as well. It was the first year both of them stayed up until midnight. They were so proud."

"Well, it's just us tonight. And while there's no cider—I do want to watch the ball go down. And to have that dance with you when it does. If you make it, that is."

"Sounds dreamy, Winnie. Wake me up just before midnight."

It is now January 1, more than an hour into a brand new year. Our dance, though short, met all expectations. It ended with a Kleenex for both of us. Nancy is in bed now, with the same relaxed look on her face as when Jayna scurried out the door. It's after midnight and we are home in our less-than-perfect apartment, without sparkling cider.

Nancy didn't ask about my favorite New Year's Eve.

The winner is *so* clear.

My favorite New Year's ever?

Tonight.

Summary: Nancy's CMV infection is under control and there isn't any "hard" evidence of GVH. So Nancy was discharged two days ago and we've returned to our Salt Lake City apartment. She is day sixty-six post-transplant, and we have only thirty-four more days before we hit the magic one-hundred-day post-transplant milestone. Our New Year's wish is to spend our days quietly in the apartment, with Nancy's health improving, and then, assuming all goes well, to return to the mountains and all our friends. And finally, I would be remiss if I didn't wish Happy New Year to you and your family.

Sincerely,

Winnie

The New Normal

January 8, 7:23 p.m.

Dear Friends and Family,

Today, there were bigger games afoot than football.

"Winnie, can you make me David and Nancy's homemade soup?"

"Boy, can I."

(Our apartment doesn't have a dishwasher—other than Jayna and me—but it does have a microwave. And soup is part of my well-known repertoire.)

"Here it is sweetheart, chicken noodle soup with lots of fixings. It smells sumptuous."

After one bite, Nancy confirmed the verdict: "Wow, this really does taste good."

By the end of the midday game, Nancy's bowl was empty. She also devoured a strawberry Carnation Instant Breakfast, made with soy milk and spiked with orange sherbet. This was the first time in our ten days on the "outside" that Nancy had eaten the equivalent of a full meal. "That cold, orange flavor not only tastes good, but it feels good on the back of my throat. Can I have some more?" It was also the first time she had asked for seconds.

The result of the nourishment? Nancy was full of energy and quite animated. After one touchdown, she screamed, "Yes!" and stood up to give Jaret a high five. She hooted and howled at two of the commercials, she whooped and shrieked at the refs, and she whooped, hollered, and grabbed my hand during the most intense moments of the game. I had not seen her so full of enthusiasm in many months.

The bowl game lasted a full five hours because of all the overtimes and commercials. Twice Nancy walked over to Jaret and Jayna, who were on the other couch, and gave each of them a hug. (She was unhooked from her IV since we had planned her medicines around this particular game.) During the postgame interviews, Nancy sneaked away from the couch and after a while, I could hear the sound of running water.

When a commercial came on, I walked into the kitchen. "Nancy, what are you doing?"

There were clean dishes in the sink and a look on Nancy's face like I had caught her with a hand in the cookie jar. "I live here too, Winnie. I get to help when I feel like it, don't I."

You have helped, my love. More than you know.

Immediately after finishing the dishes, it was time for Nancy's dressing change, Nancy's six nighttime pills, and the twelve-hour IV containing the medicine fighting Nancy's CMV infection. But for one evening, it was like old times.

"Winnie, tomorrow night can we play that board game we got for Christmas? All four of us?" (That's not a "normal" activity for our family. Rather, it's something new.)

"Sounds like fun to me," I answered, rushing to the bathroom to hide my moist eyes.

Summary: It has been a great week because it was delightfully boring and uneventful. For the first time in months, we are daring to think about tomorrow. Here's to "new" days, even ones that are not quite normal.

With love, hope and
promise,

Winnie

Sharks in the Water

January 22, 3:16 a.m.

Dear Friends and Family,

It has been pretty monotonous (and wonderful) the last two weeks. So there hasn't been much to report—that is, until my phone rang yesterday morning.

"Hello, this is Susan from the University Infusion Center. We have a delivery for Nancy Winn and want to confirm that someone's home."

"Hi, Susan. This is Nancy's husband, and unfortunately, she's at her weekly doctor's appointment. And I'm at work in Park City. What do you have for us today?"

(Supplies and medicines arrive two or three times a week at our Salt Lake City apartment. So calls like this are not unexpected and have become part of our daily routine.)

"Let's see. Heparin flushes, tubing, and some IV bags with Amphotericin"

"Excuse me, Susan, did you say Amphotericin?" (Amphotericin is a potent though highly toxic drug that combats fungal infections. Luckily, Nancy has never been required to take it. My hand went limp and I almost dropped the phone as I wondered, "Why would she need it now?")

"Yes, Mr. Winn. I did say Amphotericin. It will be in her nighttime IV. When do you expect your wife back at your apartment?"

"I'll check, Susan. And then call you back."

"Fine, let me know as soon as you find out."

My heart sank as I heard the click on the other end of the telephone line. A flurry of thoughts overwhelmed me.

Was our peaceful period over?

Does Nancy have a fungus?

A fungus could be big trouble.

By reflex, I dialed Jayna's mobile number immediately. Jayna was at the Blood and Marrow Transplant Clinic with her mother because I was at work at the clinic.

"Hey, Dadder. We're still at our appointment. We're just finishing up and talking with the doctor. Let me call you back in a couple of minutes?"

"Uh . . . all right, Jayna." I put my phone away while I replayed my conversation with Jayna over again in my mind.

Did she sound upset?

No.

Worried?

Not really.

Before I could decide what to do next, a familiar vibration jolted the area over my heart. I pulled my phone from my chest pocket. But before Jayna could even say "Hi," I blurted, "Jayna, is there something wrong with Mom? What's going on?"

"She's fine, Dadder. In fact, everyone on the team said she's doing great. They're stopping two of her pills and cutting back her nighttime IV. Why? What's the matter?"

I recounted my phone conversation with Susan. Jayna reassured me that no one had mentioned the dreaded word fungus or, for that matter, Amphotericin.

"Thanks, Jayna. You've made my day. No, my week."

I dialed the Infusion Center's number the second after I said good-bye to Jayna.

"Oh, I'm so sorry, Mr. Winn. The previous patient I talked with was the one due for Amphotericin. We don't administer that drug at home often, so it must've still been on my mind. Nancy is scheduled for Ganciclovir in her IV, not Amphotericin—just like last week. Again, I'm really sorry to have worried you."

"No problem, Susan. Nancy will be back at our apartment within the hour. I'm very happy you were wrong."

But I was unhappy that sometimes I know too much. Unfortunately, knowing too much means I am oftentimes aware of the darker possibilities and constantly looking just below the surface for any danger.

Fortunately, there weren't any sharks today.

Fortunately, there isn't any fungus either.

Summary: It has been another quiet two weeks and Nancy is making steady progress.

Love,

Winnie

A Single Blade of Grass

January 24, 12:22 p.m.

Dear Friends and Family,

"Let's go outside."

The last time I was as excited to hear those three words was when I was eight and my friend Arthur knocked on the front door of our house just after a torrential thunderstorm. The lightning and downpour ended with a rainbow that seemed to end in the woods behind my house. I jumped at the chance to go outside and search for the pot of gold. Though there was no gold to be found, we did discover a huge oak that been knocked over by the intense wind that accompanied the storm. We created a fort beneath the tree's roots that kept us entertained for the entire summer.

Today, the rainbow came from my bride. Her tooth-filled grin reflected great pride, her eyes sparkled as brilliantly as a cloudless sky in summer, and her confident attitude was more valuable to me than the pot of gold at the end of the multicolored arc. It would be our first nonhospital trip and we were venturing into the "wilds" of Salt Lake City.

Like a prisoner walking through an iron gate, Nancy looked in all directions as we slowly navigated the steps leading from the apartment. My thoughts raced ahead of us: *What is most exciting to you, my love? The jagged, snow-covered mountains in the distance? How about the shaggy stray cat that gave us a start when it darted out of the bushes to our right? Or the leafless trees revealing knobby and twisted branches only seen in the gray of winter?*

"How do things look to you, Nancy?"

"Wonderful. Everything looks wonderful."

When I made my way to the car after returning to the apartment for a mislaid wallet, Nancy was seated in the back seat of our Subaru. Jayna was firmly positioned in the front and had claimed the driver's seat.

"Nancy, you should be up front."

"Aren't people with leukemia allowed to sit in the back seat?"

Our few hours out were unadulterated joy. Observing Nancy rediscover the world was like taking a refugee back to their native country after many years away. She became animated when we rode by the house Jayna will move into when we return to the mountains—pointing out the nearby grocery store, the white wooden fence, and the single large tree in the front yard with a rope swing on its lowest branch. She recounted in great detail the many TV commercials from her hospital stays as we walked down the aisles in the grocery store. When Nancy said in a very low voice, "Ho, Ho, Ho," as we passed the Green Giant peas, Jayna almost dumped the shopping cart from a fit of laughter. Nancy stroked a fire hydrant outside the market like it was a young child, took three successive deep breaths through her nose when we entered a Starbucks coffee store, and gladly sampled five different ice creams at Baskin-Robbins before making a choice of flavors for her two scoops.

In the past, this would have been pretty unexciting stuff—but not today.

The most telling event of the afternoon happened just before we returned to the apartment. Jayna turned off the car ignition and dashed into the apartment for a "nature" call. By comparison, Nancy slowly exited our Subaru, exhausted but not in any way worse for the wear. Luckily, an old iron bench sits along the sidewalk leading to our apartment door. Nancy plopped on its wooden seat and as she turned to me said, "Just one more minute. I want to take a few more breaths of this fresh air. Can you smell the pine needles?"

Indeed, I could—but before I could answer, Nancy pointed at her feet.

"Look . . ." she exclaimed.

I didn't see anything unusual, except Nancy slipping off her left sneaker and cautiously removing the wool sock.

"What are you doing?" I asked in alarm. "You'll catch a cold." (I could hardly believe my own words, knowing that temperature has nothing to do with cold germs.) I started to laugh at myself but then realized what Nancy was doing.

"It's still alive!" she exclaimed in barely a whisper that made me wonder if she was speaking to me or just to herself.

As she talked, Nancy touched a single blade of green with her big toe. The shoot stood amid a large clump of grass colored the brown of winter. When I looked across the lawn in every direction, I saw only brown. After all, it is the end of January.

Nancy carefully put her sock and sneaker back on and extended her hand toward me. I pulled her directly into my arms and surrounded her with a huge hug. We went inside without speaking another word.

Summary: The fevers, weakness, and worries of Nancy's last hospitalization are finally fading. She surprised everyone today, wanting to venture outside the apartment. Nancy greatly enjoyed rediscovering a world she hasn't been able to be part of for a long while.

Best,

Winnie

A Shining Light

January 24, 10:44 p.m.

Dear Friends and Family,

It has been a while since I've written to you twice in one day, but today deserves and warrants a second letter.

Earlier this afternoon, when Jayna and I arrived back at the apartment, Nancy fell quickly into a deep and abiding sleep. So as not to wake Nancy, we quietly giggled for a few minutes about Nancy's grocery store antics and then I headed up the mountain to work the afternoon shift at the clinic. I had only been in my office for about twenty minutes when the phone in my pocket began vibrating. Luckily, I was not in a patient room. Jayna was on the other end.

"Hi, Dadder. You have a minute?"

In reality I didn't. I was already behind, with patients in every room.

"Sure, sweetie, what's up?"

"I just got off the phone with Delia. You remember her don't you, Dad."

"Of course, she's your best friend! How's she doing? Is she still liking Vassar?"

"More than ever, Dadder. She just got her senior thesis back. And guess what? She received a commendation—that means she's the best in her major, English."

"Wow, Jayna that's wonderful. Next time she calls, tell her I'm so happy about her achievement. And give her my congratulations."

I couldn't help but glance at the wall clock wondering, "Where is this going?" I didn't have to wait long as I almost immediately heard uncontrollable sobbing.

"Dadder, do you . . . do you think . . . do you think I would have gotten a commendation?"

I gripped the phone more tightly and ducked into the supply room. I didn't want anyone to see my face. After leaving Peru on a single day's notice, after her boyfriend was not allowed into the United States, after transferring to Utah for her senior year, Jayna was experiencing the combined weight of the world on her shoulders. All sorts of feelings from dedicating eight months of her life to our family had reached their apex and were finally coming to the surface.

"Of course, Jayna. You had a 3.9 GPA before you transferred to Utah. You have a 4.0 from your first semester here at the university. Are you missing Vassar, Jayna?"

I could hear more sobbing, which reverberated throughout my body. My heart plummeted and I immediately found that I was faulting and questioning myself.

Why couldn't I have done more?

Why had I messed up again?

Why don't I give Jayna the attention she needs?

"I'm sorry, Dadder. I shouldn't burden you."

"Jayna. I'm so sorry. I'm so very, very sorry. Your life has been turned upside down. You've had to sacrifice so much. I wish that your mother and I had been more insistent that you go back to Vassar. I wish you were there right now . . ."

Jayna didn't respond for what seemed like a long time. When she did, she had regained her composure: "It's all right, Dadder. Mom means more than anything else. It was just hard for a moment."

I bet it was, my sweet, sweet daughter. You've been incredibly strong and incredibly helpful. You have been a shining light to your mother during the darkest times. You're able to make her laugh when there was little reason for laughter.

"Hey, Jayna. I'll tell you what. Let's go out and celebrate— for Delia and for you."

"That would be great, Dadder."

Life is slowly getting back to normal in the Winn household. We are starting to reflect on the past—and even daring to contemplate the future. The fog of Nancy's disease is slowly lifting. It is a happier time for us. But there is a toll paid by the family of anyone with a chronic or life-threatening disease.

"Jayna, consider this. The fact you're thinking about Vassar means Mom is really getting better. I'll see you in a few hours when I get off work. We'll tuck Mom in and then go raise a glass to Delia, you, and Mom."

And, of course, to all of you.

Summary: Day eighty-nine post-transplant and counting. We are three and a half weeks out of the hospital now. Most days are blissfully unexciting. On some days, Nancy barely gets out of bed; others are without a single nap. We watch a lot of TV together, and the other day, there was even a novel on Nancy's nightstand. Nancy is tolerating full meals regularly. She continues to take baby steps toward recovery. The result of Nancy's increasing recovery is that Jayna is also looking outward at what, until now, has been all but impossible.

As always,

Winnie

An Age-Old Ritual

January 29, 11:45 p.m.

Dear Friends and Family,

Early this morning, I found myself hesitantly standing outside the door of our apartment's bedroom so as not to disturb a tableau-like moment that was being shared between Nancy and Jayna. My "two girls," framed by the doorway, were talking to the full-length mirror. They would point at the mirror and then Jayna would turn her mother 180 degrees. I heard only laughter and delight as Nancy strained her neck to glimpse at her image. Then, unexpectedly, Jayna walked away and returned with a hat in her hand.

"I like the red one!" Jayna exclaimed, as she angled the hat so its low side nearly hid Nancy's left ear. "It will be a fashion statement and it matches your new red top."

"What about this dark-blue one?" Nancy asked, pulling a round hat with a larger brim from the pile of wigs, scarves, and head coverings spread across the entirety of the queen bed.

"This one looks great, too. It could work with your navy top. Both go with your black pants or these new jeans." Jayna held the denim slacks in front of Nancy while both posed in front of the mirror. "Put them on, Mommer."

Mothers and daughters choosing an outfit—it's an age-old ritual that used to drive me nuts. Today, however, it brings tears to my eyes because Nancy is getting ready for a special occasion.

Despite my effort to be quiet and invisible, Jayna noticed me in the doorway. "Dadder, doesn't this look good on Mom? Which shirt do you like best?" Jayna holds first the red and then the blue blouse in front of Nancy.

I look for a place to hide. To me, everything looks good.

"Jayna, you know better. Your father is clothing 'challenged.' Just put both in my suitcase. We'll make a final decision later."

Nancy really means "Jayna's" suitcase. It's the only luggage residing in our Salt Lake City apartment. Jayna purchased the valise for twenty dollars in Peru when she hastily returned to the United States. The suitcase's exterior is green paisley and it had been large enough for Jayna to throw everything in it when she made her mad dash to the airport.

"That's too big. We're only going for one night," I had been laughingly admonished by Jayna.

Now it's a different story. My pajamas probably won't fit and there may not be room for my toothbrush—especially since Nancy and Jayna continue to hunt for the "right" combination.

Jayna winks. "You may have to use a Toys 'R' Us bag for your stuff, Dadder. I saw one under the sink in the kitchen. Jaret won't mind."

I retreat to the kitchen to retrieve the sack, with the continuing sounds of cheerful banter in my ear. The celebration has already been a huge success and we're not even in Park City yet for our dinner in a real restaurant.

Celebration?

Dinner in Park City?

A real restaurant?

Yes.

Although tonight is still several days before the magical one-hundred-day post-transplant target, two of Nancy's dearest friends arrived yesterday.

So why not celebrate early?

What could be more appropriate than an unexpected return to the mountains?

What could be more fun than a slumber party at Emmy and Fred's house?

A night out is mundane if you don't have leukemia. A meal at a favorite restaurant might even seem routine if you don't have leukemia. For us, however, food from a printed menu served by a waitress is an all-but-forgotten luxury. (Our last visit to Ghidotti's, Nancy's favorite restaurant in Park City, was the night before her transplant hospitalization in October. At the time, we wondered if Nancy would ever eat in a restaurant again.)

At dinner tonight, Nancy only tolerated one sip of wine—her taste buds are still not yet ready for more of the "nectar of the gods." But the food was delicious and she consumed nearly a full portion of linguini with white clam sauce, a dish she longed for during her many months of nausea. Dinner was a delight and a triumph in equal measures. Just weeks ago, a single spoonful was considered a meal by Nancy.

In the center of our table, there was a flickering candle that sent soft shadows across the fine crystal, elegant silverware, and uniquely shaped dishes. The lighted taper illuminated Nancy's face. Her blue eyes, highlighted by the blue hat, were filled with joy and jubilant luster.

I watched Nancy like a mother hen for signs of fatigue, but it was Jaret who commanded her full attention when he described his college classes to Lyn, Nancy's friend from Marblehead, Massachusetts. There were no heavy eyelids tonight. Nancy even told us about flying into Las Vegas during the "old days" with John, our other out-of-town guest, from Salem, Massachusetts. Lyn and John both flew with Nancy when she worked for TWA. Nancy introduced them to me years ago and they quickly became my friends, too.

Nancy is so much stronger this past week. Her giggle almost reached the table next to us and her smile seemed wider tonight too—especially when she tasted Jayna's fettuccine alfredo and sneaked a bite of Fred and Emmy's clams casino.

This evening, chills raced down my arms when I realized that I haven't seen Nancy look this good for a long, long time. There are now fewer wrinkles on Nancy's forehead, her shoulders sit higher than last week, and she exudes warmth and beauty.

For a moment, I wondered if it was the hat?

But in reality, I know the real answer.

Summary: Two of Nancy's best friends from her TWA flying days are visiting from Boston. So we turned the evening into an early one-hundred-day post-transplant celebration by going to one of her favorite restaurants in Park City and then having a "sleepover" in the mountain home of Emmy and Fred. Life is good—very good.

With much love,

Winnie

The Mother of Good Fortune

February 7, 10:56 p.m.

Dear Friends and Family,

Nancy has spent the past three days uneventfully staying up into the wee hours, watching sitcoms with Jayna, reading about social anthropology with Jaret for one of his last college courses, and eating several meals regularly—though not as flamboyantly as at Ghidotti's.

All in all, Nancy had continued to do well as we approached day one hundred.

On day ninety-seven after her bone marrow transplant, we returned to the hospital for a regularly scheduled visit. For a full day, we felt like we were school children scurrying from class to class as we completed the many parts of Nancy's "one-hundred-day evaluation." (The one-hundred-day evaluation is an intense look at how a patient's body has tolerated the many medicines received during the bone marrow transplant process. The critical question is, "Have the many pills and IV medicines caused any damage?")

We started our sessions with the hospital dentist, who closely scrutinized Nancy's teeth and gums; moved on to the pulmonary function lab to check the health of Nancy's lungs; and then headed to the hospital outpatient lab for a "gazillion" blood tests. We next traveled to the transplant lab where a skin biopsy was performed and they did an eye tear-making challenge test that would look for low-grade graft-versus-host disease.

Later in the day, Nancy underwent her first bone marrow test since the transplant to examine how the donor cells were "enjoying" their new home and to be certain there were no traces of leukemia. She also received a chest X-ray and an EKG and saw a gynecologist. It was a full day—to say the least.

Quite honestly, we were nervous as she went from office to office. At each stop there was a test. A passing grade was vital.

"Winnie, when you tell people I'm feeling good, it's all relative. I definitely feel light years better compared to when I first got sick. I'm considerably improved especially when I think of how tired I was after the transplant. But I'm far from normal yet."

As I listened intently to Nancy, I couldn't help but think to myself: *How well I know, my love. But I have seen hints this past week that you are gaining strength.*

"I'm not complaining. I just don't want our friends to think I'm ready to go out every night. I don't want them to wonder why I may not have written back or returned calls."

"I understand, Nancy," I said out loud this time. "I think they do, too, but I'll do better. I'll tell them you're a three or a four."

We both enjoyed my "inside" joke. (Nancy is constantly asked to quantify her continuing leg pain on a one-to-ten scale. She always answers "a three or a four," but we jest about her saying "twenty-five" or "minus seven" to see what kind of response she is able to provoke.)

Our conversation was interrupted as we entered the Blood and Marrow Transplant Clinic where Nancy would have the all-important bone marrow test. Laurie, the nurse, gave Nancy a hug and asked about the kids and Katie, the clerk, walked over to greet us. "It's good to see you, Nancy. Have you enjoyed your time at the apartment?" Before Nancy could answer, Carly, the medical assistant checking in Nancy, frowned after reading the thermometer she had just removed from Nancy's left ear. She quickly grabbed a different thermometer and tested Nancy's right ear again.

"You did tell me you're feeling good didn't you, Nancy? You haven't had a cough or diarrhea?"

Nancy shook her head, and I dropped mine lower.

"Well, Nancy, it appears you have a fever. 101.5 degrees. Let me get Malinda."

Malinda was the nurse practitioner in charge of the clinic. By the time she arrived, Nancy's temperature had been retaken in both ears, plus a glass thermometer was placed under her tongue. Each thermometer registered similar values. Elevated—averaging 101.6. Melinda reviewed the history, listened to Nancy's lungs, and immediately ordered more tests.

I sat somewhat in a daze and stupor. I understood and followed each step being taken by the medical staff, but it still felt dreamlike and surreal. (No, actually it felt more like a nightmare.) I placed the back of my hand on Nancy's forehead and was given the answer directly. Nancy felt hot. The thermometers were accurate.

"I'm sorry, Nancy and Winnie. To be safe, we'll need to put you back in the hospital. You look so good, too. It should be a short visit."

Did we celebrate one hundred days too early?

Is this the beginning of a serious infection?

How many steps backward have we taken this time?

Numerous questions raced through my mind as we waited twenty-four hours. Fortunately, a culture of Nancy's blood revealed that she had a bacterium—staph.

"Isn't the staph germ the one that kills people, Dr. Ford?"

Not the question I wanted her to ask, but that's Nancy—ever straightforward.

"There are many different types of staph, Nancy. You have a common one that lives on the skin and, in all likelihood, contaminated your central IV line. We caught it really early, even before you had symptoms. I think it will be easy to treat."

We were fortunate this week.

Yesterday, after only two days on the fifth floor of University of Utah Hospital, Nancy returned home to our apartment. We didn't decorate her hospital room this time, and Jayna didn't sleep there a single night. (I did, however.) Nancy is back on antibiotics into a new IV site, but she continues to feel good.

As we were leaving the hospital, she whispered, "At least a three or four," in my ear as we exited into the sunshine and fresh air. Our brief hospital stay serves as a reminder that Nancy was very sick in the past (twenty-five on the one-to-ten scale) and that, even now, she remains fragile. Although today marks exactly one hundred days from the transplant, our journey is far from over.

So what happens on day one hundred?

Day one hundred is a significant milestone. Twenty percent of patients with Nancy's condition don't make it to day one hundred. Nancy's brush with a systemic infection three days ago is a brutal reminder. I try not to dwell on what could have happened. We are so blessed to have had a coincidental hospital appointment. For once, luck was on our side.

Obstacles can still arise at the snap of a finger. So we will enjoy today to the fullest, as well as every other day that Nancy feels better than a "three" or "four." But we have to remain ever vigilant.

Next week, after all the blood work and tests are completed, we will visit with Dr. Peterson to learn the post-one-hundred-day landscape. We already know Nancy will begin six months of decreasing medicine intake. The less her bone marrow is suppressed, the more it can protect against staph and other germs. It will be a balancing act, because more freedom means increased risk of graft-versus-host problems. But an end will be in sight, with the mountains in our future.

Upon reflection, we'll postpone the fireworks today.

Instead we will meditate on where we were, how good things are now, and what's truly important—friends and family.

Summary: Three days ago was Nancy's day one hundred post-transplant. Day one hundred is a significant milestone for any bone marrow transplant patient. Day one hundred signifies that Nancy's "baby steps" toward recovery are finally adding up. Nancy has undergone multiple tests to see how her body's organs have fared, and we haven't gotten any alarming results. It is particularly exciting given that Nancy had another two-day hospital stay earlier in the week that was unscheduled and unexpected. Fortunately, she is celebrating this milestone at home and feeling decent.

All my love,

Winnie

Thoughts on Kissing a Fashionista

February 18, 6:21 p.m.

Dear Friends and Family,

The last time we were required to come to the hospital, Nancy was appearing to have a seemingly healthy day. She had increased strength, improved appetite, and less leg pain. We were absolutely shocked when it was discovered she had a fever. And frankly, it was very depressing and frightening when she was readmitted to the fifth floor. Luckily, Nancy's hospitalization lasted only two days because the infection had just started and was caused by a germ easily treated by antibiotics.

It is not surprising, then, that as I dropped Nancy off at the hospital's front door today and left to park the car, my stomach started to stir uneasily again. The "fifth floor" windows of our last three rooms were all clearly visible to me as I walked from the parking lot back to the hospital. For this reason, I suspect that I will always feel somewhat unsettled when I pass through the revolving hospital doors. (In reality, it actually sucks that I require antacids when I bring Nancy to the hospital.).

This time, however, the appointment went smoothly. Not only did Nancy look and feel healthy, her exam (including her temperature) was normal.

"Do you have any questions?" asked the physician assistant, Robert.

"Yes, we were just wondering if any of Nancy's tests are back. We were told the bone marrow exam might be done by today."

As we waited for a response to our question, I found myself for some unknown reason thinking about "kissing."

My first kiss with someone other than a "relative" occurred when I was nine years old. Her name was Andrea, and she had a long, blonde ponytail and lots of freckles. I was at summer camp. We only kissed that one time, and I never saw her again after we returned to our separate homes.

I didn't experience the same butterflies in my stomach and tingling in my toes again until I was thirty. It was the first time I kissed Nancy and I was saying good-bye to her in Yellowstone National Park. I remember our kiss as it if it was yesterday, and I also distinctly recollect wondering if I would ever see her again.

Nancy, in fact, did come back to Yellowstone the next week, and by the fifth time we kissed, it was comfortable and fulfilling, sentiments that have remained unchanged for the last twenty-eight years.

Bone marrow tests are different from kisses, though.

As I waited for the test results for the fifth time, it was no less frightening, no less easy, and certainly no less important. Robert left the room for two, maybe three, minutes. Time stood still and each of those minutes was an eternity.

My wait was exactly like the first time.

And the second.

And the third.

And the fourth.

Nancy, on the other hand, barely noticed Robert's absence. Her face, unlike mine, was content, playful, and happy. She busied herself interacting with the TV remote, changing the channels, and adjusting the picture and sound. (I'm certain it felt good for her to control something. For months at a time, she was too weak to even hold a remote.)

Robert knocked as he reentered the room. Nancy accurately hit the mute button and said with a smile, "You're back." The next few seconds were agonizingly long. I searched for a hint in his eyes, his face, or even in his body language. Before I could find a clue, Robert handed me three sheets of lab results as he addressed my better half.

"Well, Nancy, it's a clean sweep. Congratulations! Your bone marrow is perfect. No leukemia. And your skin biopsy shows no sign of graft-versus-host disease."

Robert discussed the other more routine lab work, but I tuned him out. I bit my lower lip and concentrated. Don't break down, Winnie, I told myself. Nancy glanced my way and smiled, then nodded her head up and down ever so slightly. She knew. She grabbed my hand and put it between both of hers.

My bride. You are so much stronger than me.

"So," Robert finished, "You will hear from Rachael later in the day about your meeting with Dr. Peterson. He will map out the next steps. Again, congratulations to you both. Oh, and . . . I love your shirt and scarf."

Nancy and I were both wearing T-shirts that we had received special delivery from her childhood friends in Calhoun, Georgia—Tes, Can, Nita, and Bootie. "Happy 100th Day," the shirts read on the front and "We're always behind you" was written across the back. In addition, in keeping with her "fashionista" approach to her personal attire, Nancy's head covering was also distinctive. It was a "buff" from *Survivor*, a present from Emmy and our Christmas angel's husband, Fred, which prominently displayed the reality TV show's title.

Today, all things being equal, both Nancy's shirt and head covering were very fitting.

Summary: Nancy's test results confirm that she has met the biggest challenge of a bone marrow transplant patient older than twenty. She is leukemia-free at the one-hundred-day post-transplant milestone.

Best,

Winnie

The Real Deal

February 24, 1:00 a.m.

Dear Friends and Family,

You may not be aware, but my partners and I provide both weekend and extended hours to our community because the nearest hospital and emergency room is a half-hour drive away in Salt Lake City. Many of the shifts I work at the clinic end late in the evening because we offer a place for Park City residents and guests to obtain medical care and treatment during nontraditional hours.

After work tonight, I raced through the door of the clinic at 8:05 p.m., eager to "get down the canyon" to our apartment. Though I've been commuting to Salt Lake City for almost nine months, I still find the drive difficult. The lion's share of the commute is on Interstate 80, over a mountain pass and through a narrow canyon. The drive, more often than not, is often a white-knuckle adventure.

Almost always, in addition to the reoccurring curves, there are lots of speeding semitrailer trucks and "big rigs"—plus snow in the winter as I speed (not literally) to our "home" away from home. But not tonight. There were very few cars on the road, and a brilliant full moon lit my entire way to Nancy. In the back of my mind was the thought that if I arrived by 9:00 p.m., there would be a quality hour with Nancy before bed. I pulled into the apartment parking lot at 8:47 p.m., daydreaming about our old (but functional) couch. My feet were up, Nancy's head was on my lap, and I was holding her hand ever so lightly. All things considered, it would be an appropriate end to a long day.

"Hi, Winnie, how are you?" Nancy's toe-tingling kiss erased the chill from my lips as I walked through the door. I immediately thought to myself that at this time of night, she usually doesn't have the strength to meet me at the door.

I choked on the word "tired" and changed it to "fine."

As my eyes slowly focused to the lower light in the apartment, I noticed that Nancy was dressed in clothes—not PJs. She had on her *Survivor* "buff" head covering.

"Guess what, Winnie? Michaela from ASA called. My friends are having a party, starting at nine. If you hurry, we'll be hardly more than fashionably late."

"All right, dear." (What else could I possibly say as I gazed longingly at the couch?)

We only stayed an hour, but Nancy was the guest of honor of some of her flying colleagues before her illness. When we arrived, I placed her on a couch with her feet up, kept the host's cat away, and made sure that she didn't partake of the vodka, gin, and other libations there were readily available. But it was a real party—nonetheless.

"Thanks for taking me, Winnie. It meant a lot to me."

And to them, my love.

Summary: Nancy went to her first real party this evening. I hope it is the first of many and that she will feel up to raising a glass with each of you in the near future.

All our best,

Winnie

The Best Gift of All

February 26, 7:03 p.m.

Dear Friends and Family,

When Dr. Finn Bo Peterson visited us at LDS Hospital last year on August 12, Nancy was completing her second round of chemotherapy. The news was not favorable. *"If Nancy doesn't have a transplant, she has a 5–10% chance of long-term survival—at best."* As you well know, his words were both devastating and demoralizing. At the time, we thought Nancy had an even 50/50 chance for survival. We were thrust into a different reality and had to make many hard decisions.

Today, more than six and a half months after that very dark day, we met again with Finn Bo. This time, the news was different. Our meeting couldn't have been more dissimilar, too. It was the difference between night and day.

"I am really pleased with your progress, Nancy. I know it has been a long and difficult road, but you have made it. And I am optimistic you will continue to do well."

Finn Bo discussed each of Nancy's results. We already knew the most important one, her bone marrow test. It is normal and there is no evidence of leukemia.

"Have any of Nancy's organs shown the trauma of her treatments, Dr. Petersen?" I asked.

"Winnie, the only question mark is her lungs. Nancy had a chest X-ray that was perfectly fine, but one of her lung function tests was decreased compared with the same test before the transplant. It's not dangerous or worrisome. But we'll want to repeat the test when we do her next bone marrow again, in three months. On the good side, her liver and kidney function are both great, and her new marrow is producing plenty of white cells, red cells, and platelets. So we can begin tapering Nancy's immunosuppressing drug, Cyclosporine, today. It should take about six months."

"What will that do, Dr. Peterson?" Nancy inquired.

"You may remember, Nancy, that Cyclosporine is the drug that's kept your graft in check to allow it to ease into your body. But now's the time for your transplanted marrow to gain full strength."

"What things do we need to worry about in this next phase?"

"Our major concerns are pretty much the same, Winnie. Infection and GVH (graft-versus-host disease). As the graft is unleashed, the risk of infection will drop—but the chance of GVH will be increased."

"What are the numbers now for contracting GVH and, more importantly, Nancy's long-term chances? And what is the 'long term' in Nancy's disease?"

(I felt so stupid. I know better. One should never ask more than a single question at a time.)

"Well, with Nancy making it through these difficult one hundred days, we adjust the curves. Nancy now has only a 20–30% chance of developing GVH. And I think her chance of cure, of being disease-free at two years after transplant, is as high as 75–80%."

(Remember, before the transplant, we were told Nancy had about a 75% chance of developing GVH. And only a 50% chance of survival.)

"Wow, Dr. Peterson! I love the new numbers. Thanks, I don't have any more questions."

I glanced at Nancy. She was beaming and her face lit up with the biggest of smiles.

And me?

As is my tendency, I was struggling to put corks in my tear ducts until after the meeting. Nancy never turned my way, but instead, she grabbed my hand just like always. And, no surprise to me, she pivoted immediately to the practical.

"When can I go to Park City?"

"What about Woodland?"

"Can I drive?"

"Can I be alone for more than a minute?"

"How about out-of-state travel?"

Dr. Peterson patiently answered each and every one of Nancy's questions. Technically, her leash was "lengthened" logarithmically. We have been cleared to live in Park City by March 1. She can reclaim her car (while we stay at the Marshalls' home) from Jayna—but no plane or car trips until fall. Notably, our most cherished dream is also now close enough to touch.

We will be home to Woodland by April.

Sooner than we can imagine, we'll be entertaining—you.

Summary: Nancy passed her one-hundred-day post-transplant evaluation with flying colors. We will return to the mountains soon, barring any setbacks. And today is my birthday. I couldn't have asked for a better present.

Fondly,

Winnie

The Good, the Bad, and *the Ugly*

March 11, 3:48 a.m.

Dear Friends and Family,

In my last update, I consciously tried to avoid euphoria while reporting Nancy's incredible day one-hundred post-transplant test results.

Quite honestly, when I heard "a 75–80% chance" tied to the sacred word cure, I wanted to believe with every fiber in my being that we truly are "on our way" to a normal life. After nine and a half months of repeated struggles, Nancy's news feels leap years better than good.

I must admit that it wasn't that long ago that I was overcome by depression when I heard bad numbers early in our battle. As a result, my spirit is somewhat tempered by the several times I have wondered if we were facing the end. Somehow, I knew that with a long stretch of road still ahead—more bumps were likely.

Last night, after Nancy fell asleep, in an effort to stop my mind from racing, I rewatched a movie called *Million Dollar Baby*, directed by and starring Clint Eastwood. The title caught my attention because it made me think of the expense of Nancy's treatment. It is something I purposely have avoided thinking about. Fortunately, Nancy is doubly covered by two fully comprehensive insurances. Undoubtedly, our family has been extremely lucky.

As I watched my movie, I recalled other films by Eastwood. Some of you are old enough to remember one of his first big successes, *The Good, the Bad, and the Ugly*. Justifiably, that title is the perfect description of Nancy's recent encounters with her vital central IV line. So let me begin my story anew by using Eastwood's title. (But in this instance, I'll emphasize only part of his title.)

I'll call my story, *"The Ugly."*

"Dad, there's a pool of blood in the dining room. Mom's PICC line fell out."

After a hard day's work, driving to Salt Lake City sometimes requires maximum concentration. However, when I received a distressed call from Jayna, I almost ran off the road before my medical training clicked in and I responded in a calm voice, *"Jayna, are you saying Mom's IV line pulled out of her arm?"*

"Yes."

"And that she's bleeding from the site?"

"Yes."

"Is she still conscious and alert?"

"Yes she is, Dadder."

"Are you putting pressure on the area?"

"Uh huh."

"Has the bleeding stopped?"

"I think so. We used almost an entire roll of paper towels. I'm squeezing her arm with both hands and holding it up above her head. The blood isn't dripping anymore."

"Sounds like you've done all the right things, Jayna. How is Mom feeling?"

"She's hungry. She's excited to eat the Chinese meal that just arrived. We ordered takeout."

"That is encouraging, Jayna. Do you have Mom lying down?"

"No. She is insistent that she sits in a chair. You know Mommer."

"Great job, Jayna. I'm just passing Lamb's Canyon so I'm about fifteen minutes away from you. Do you think we need to call 911?"

"I don't think so, Dadder. I'd rather wait 'til you get here. All right?"

"Only if you're sure Mom's bleeding has stopped. Is she dizzy or complaining of anything else? Where's Jaret?"

"He's cleaning the floor. Can you believe it?"

No, I can't.

(As most of you may know already before Nancy's illness, Jaret wouldn't even talk about blood, let alone get near it.)

As I raced to get to the apartment, I found myself thinking that I couldn't believe any of this was happening. Just when I expected to cruise along, to begin enjoying life, Nancy grew germs from the IV line in her chest—the one that enters her central circulation through the large vein beneath her clavicle. It's scary, knowing a bug was living in her blood, a silent assassin waiting quietly to strike. After eight hours in the hospital, that particular IV line (and the germs on its tip) was gone. The team carefully placed a new one, in her right arm and now, and just a few weeks later, it gets accidentally pulled out.

"Jayna, if anything changes, if Mom gets dizzy or the bleeding starts up again or anything else, call the ambulance immediately—then me."

By the time I arrived at the apartment, I was second-guessing myself.

Should I have insisted Jayna call 911?

Could we have prevented this somehow?

Did I tell Jayna and Jaret how well they reacted?

And the biggest question, how is Nancy doing?

My answer came quickly. As I rushed through the door, heart racing and legs wobbly, there was Nancy sitting nonchalantly at the table in the dining room. Her right upper arm, the one that had formerly contained the IV, was wrapped in paper towels. In turn, Jayna was firmly holding Nancy's arm in her two hands. At the same time, Nancy's free left arm was quite busy as she scooped bite after bite of a variety of Chinese delicacies into her mouth from an endless array of square white cardboard containers spread across the table.

"Hey, Winnie, what's happening? Sit. Sit. You look harried. You probably need an egg roll before we head to the hospital."

There was no choice. I burst into laughter as I watched Nancy savoring each and every spoonful of Chinese takeout. She was the picture of calm, a stark contrast to Jaret and Jayna standing on either side of her looking like they were watching *Friday the 13th.*

"I can't figure out what happened, Winnie. My line was clipped to my pajamas like always. All I did was take off my robe so I could eat. Gremlins must have yanked it out."

Nancy's message was obvious. No worries here, Winnie.

"I'll take that egg roll, Nancy. Actually, give me two."

Summary: We continue to joke our way through challenges whenever possible. When Nancy accidentally pulled out her IV eleven days ago and bled all over the apartment, we were given just such an opportunity.

Warmly,

Winnie

The Good, *the Bad,* and the Ugly

March 12, 5:32 a.m.

Dear Friends and Family,

As promised yesterday, I will now continue with my story titled *"The Bad."*

Two days after the Chinese takeout blood bath, we seemed to be back on the right path. Nancy sported yet another new IV, this time higher up in her right arm. We began preparing for our move to the mountains. We were also enjoying a visit with Linda, Nancy's sister from Atlanta.

Thinking it would be a quick and routine visit, Linda took Nancy to her early weekly doctor's appointment. (Jayna and I slept in, taking the morning off.) Unfortunately, I didn't get to sleep long, as my phone rang at about 8:30 a.m. "Hey, Winnie. It's Linda. Renae, the nurse practitioner at the clinic today, wants to know if you did something different this morning when you drew Nancy's blood."

Though I did go back to sleep, that was only after drawing Nancy's labs before she went to the hospital. Since it saves time, I have become the "phlebotomist" as part of our daily routine.

"No, I don't think so. What's wrong?"

"Nancy's hematocrit came back low—20%."

"You're kidding. That's not low, that's extremely low. It's never been 20%, even when she was unable to make her own red cells. In fact, they gave her blood transfusions whenever it dipped below 24%."

"They're rechecking it right now. If it comes back the same, she'll be given blood immediately. I'll call back as soon as we hear something. Also, Nancy says to stop worrying—and to not wake Jayna up or say anything to her when she does get up."

The next hour was filled with gloomy thoughts and a queasy nervousness. As I paced the floor, I wondered: Could Nancy have lost that much blood when her IV came out two days ago? Did I screw up when I was drawing the labs this morning? (The only other likely causes I could think of were disasters— like, "I'm sorry, Winnie. Nancy's leukemia is back.")

Practically, I hoped for a blood draw "snafu." I wished that the recheck of her blood count would weigh in around 30%, lower than the 42% for the general public—but "normal" for Nancy. I searched for clues like a detective. I even examined the materials that I had put in the trash. I retraced every step from the entire morning looking for blood on the floor. And not surprising, I thought about Nancy and our future.

Yesterday, Nancy was tired. Still, she did homework with Jaret for over seven hours. I had been exhausted just watching. Nancy hadn't worked like that since before her first hospitalization. I rationalized that her hematocrit couldn't be 20%. Nancy would have fallen asleep by simply walking to the bathroom. Even simple things, like brushing her teeth, would have required too much effort. Yesterday, when Jaret proudly displayed his finished paper, Nancy's smile matched Jaret's. Neither of them appeared exhausted. The low number had to be from something I did.

Finally the phone rang. "It wasn't you, Winnie. The redraw confirmed Nancy's hematocrit—20.4%. We'll be here a while. They've ordered two units of blood STAT. For so few red cells, they can't believe how good she looks."

Summary: Even this far removed from her transplant, we are reminded once again that Nancy's health is fragile.

With love,

Winnie

The Good, the Bad, and the Ugly

March 12, 9:18 p.m.

Dear Friends and Family,

When I wrote you this morning, I got so emotional that I sent my note before I shared the last part of my trilogy.

So, here is "*The Good*."

After a week had passed following the low blood count episode, I kissed Nancy's fuzzy head at ten o'clock one morning, an hour earlier than our most recent custom, and said quietly, "Wake up beautiful, it's time to get ready. I need to borrow some blood."

"Borrow?"

On the ride to the hospital for her follow-up appointment, I wondered what would happen this time. Nancy's serenity didn't extend to my side of the car. She grabbed my hand. "Today will be a good day, Winnie. Don't worry."

Her eyes sparkled so intensely I partially swerved onto the shoulder for a moment. "Relax," she commanded. "And try not to hit anybody."

How does Nancy always sense my feelings? And soothe them.

Predictably, Nancy was right again. When Malinda, our nurse practitioner, knocked on the exam room door and walked into the room, her eyebrows were raised and she immediately shook both our hands. "Your labs are perfect, Nancy. You are finally drinking and eating enough. And the best part is that your blood cultures are negative. The bug is gone. There's no more need for IV antibiotics. You know what that means?"

With a controlled pull and immediate pressure, Nancy's IV line was removed. Her constant companion came painlessly out of her arm, and there was less than a drop of blood lost.

"There," Malinda said as she threw the tubing into the red garbage can designated for medical waste and took off her gloves. "How long has it been, Nancy?"

"Let's see. I've had one IV or another most of the time since my first admission—I guess that was May 29. I can't even remember what it's going to be like to take a shower without it. I always had to worry about getting the site wet and causing another infection."

The good, the bad, and the ugly.

For over nine months now, Nancy has crawled, limped, or charged through the bad and the ugly to reach the good. The day after her IV was removed, we packed our belongings and left Salt Lake City for our return to the mountains. We had barely walked through the door of the Marshalls' home, where we were to spend the next month, when Nancy shed her clothes and raced into the shower of their master bedroom.

"You all right, Nancy? You've been in there a long time."

All I heard was a guttural sound: "Ahhh!"

Through the fog-covered glass of the shower door, I could see that Nancy's entire body was adorned in soap. Water streamed down her face and jumped from the edges of her mouth. Her lips were widely separated and her pearly whites dazzling despite the increasing steam that was rapidly engulfing the bathroom.

She is amazing.

And I could also hear Nancy's uplifting laughter and see her beautiful smile beneath the water streaming off the tip of her nose on to the bathroom tile below.

Summary: The last few weeks have been a time of guarded triumph tempered with a dose of reality. Generally, our path has been upward, figuratively and literally. After all, this week we returned to our beloved mountains. For the next month, we will be living in our friend's home in Pinebrook, a housing development just over Parley's Summit. Our friends, the Marshalls, are vacationing in Florida for the month of March and they have graciously offered us their home with its ever-present warmth. The Marshalls' home is a wonderful intermediary stop on our journey back to Woodland and is within easy striking distance to the hospital—if needed.

Much love and thanks,

Winnie

This Isn't Our First Rodeo

March 24, 6:46 p.m.

Dear Friends and Family,

When Nancy awoke one morning last week, her report was not favorable.

"Winnie, I just don't feel right. I'm not hungry—even water tastes bad. All I want to do is sleep. What does it mean?"

The previous four days had seen a gradual decline in our "vacation." Each night after work, we still talked and relaxed by a roaring fire. Fortunately, Nancy could still stay awake for the final credits of the video I rented each day—but there were no more trips to the market, no visits to the nearby outlet mall, and no back-booth, off-hours restaurant meals. In fact, Nancy's oral intake had become an increasing concern.

"Are you nauseated, Nancy?"

"Had any cramping?"

"How about vomiting or diarrhea?"

Each of Nancy's replies was an unpleasant shock to me.

"Actually, yes . . . I didn't want you to worry, Winnie. I didn't think it was a big deal."

I knew differently.

"We need to call the transplant team, Nancy."

By that afternoon, Nancy was readmitted to University of Utah Hospital, and the elevator ride to the Fifth Floor was once again filled with unpleasant memories. I was sad, devastated, and even frightened, too.

"Everything's fine, Winnie. I'll feel much better once I'm rehydrated. And a PICC (central IV) line isn't so bad. It will help us get home sooner. This isn't our first rodeo."

How does she do it?

We were so close—a week away from our Woodland home. We had discussed our first meal there, our first visitors, and our first walk by the river.

Thankfully, the medical team quickly discovered a treatable GI bug. Once again, there is no evidence of graft-versus-host disease on the small bowel biopsy. In return, Nancy gave up the freedom of an IV-free shower, but we were able to return to the Marshalls' home in Park City seven days later.

Once again, Nancy was right.

Summary: We continue to take one step back for every two steps forward. This time, our "backward" step included a week's stay in the hospital fighting yet another GI bug. We cannot wait for Nancy's new immune system to gain full strength.

Best,

Winnie

The Best Laid Plans

March 31, 7:04 p.m.

Dear Friends and Family,

Nancy has lots of books. Before her illness, a paperback was almost always in Nancy's delicate hands or close by on the nightstand. Unfortunately, our home has only so many tables and so many niches. Our single small bookcase has always resembled my stomach after Thanksgiving dinner—too full.

All that changed today, March 31.

"Well, Nancy, how does it look to you?"

I opened the front door to Woodland for Nancy and waved my hand like a bellman as she walked into our home. Her steps were confident and her smile filled her face. As she entered the mud room, she clapped her hands and I heard a playful giggle.

(Today wasn't April 1 and it certainly was no joke. For me, it was a combination of Thanksgiving, my birthday, and the spring season's first mountain bike ride—all wrapped into one.)

The last time Nancy passed through the door to our home was 156 days ago. Five months, two weeks, and one day exactly. After Nancy left for her transplant hospitalization on October 17, she had never returned to our mountain dream home. I could only imagine what it must be like for her. My palms were sweaty like on our first date, and Nancy's eyes darted in all directions, taking in all that was familiar.

"Everything looks fantastic, Winnie. I can tell the cleaners were here this morning. It even smells clean."

(I momentarily considered telling Nancy that "the cleaners" were two of her dedicated friends, Janis and Joannie, rather than hired professionals but chose not to as attention of this sort is hard for my Nancy.)

"And the windows sparkle? You got them washed, didn't you?"

(Indeed. I did. It's worth every penny to see your eyes sparkle even more than the glass.)

"And look at the plants. They made it! I'm so surprised."

(Me too. One of many things I've learned during your illness, Nancy. I actually now know how to water a plant—not too little and not too much.)

Nancy walked to the edge of the living room and made a loud sigh of contentment and relief. For several minutes, she gazed at the river and trees through the full-length windows. Both the lawn and the aspen trees were frosted with a new coating of snow tinged with the slightest hint of orange, a reflection of the impending sunset.

As she returned to me on the other side of the room, Nancy touched the back of a chair, straightened a book on the coffee table next to the couch, and ran her hand over the soft comforter draped on the back of the recliner. She gestured to the Christmas tree and laughed softly. The twinkle of the tree lights stood out brightly for her homecoming. She didn't have to ask because she knew already that for me, today was better than Christmas.

"I think I might take a nap," Nancy mumbled as she began to move slowly toward the bedroom.

"Can you believe what everyone did along the road on the way to the house?"

"How many 'Welcome Home' signs were there between Francis and Woodland?"

"Who brought the balloons and put the food in the refrigerator?"

"The banner over the front door was professionally made, wasn't it?"

"Not to worry now, Nancy. We'll thank each member of your 'welcoming' committee in good time. They love you, Nancy, and they had so much fun. You have so many friends." I caressed and touched her arm ever so lightly. "I can't figure out why."

Nancy wrapped her arms tightly around me. A real kiss warmed my lips and a familiar tingle reached my toes.

"Sweetie, you need your rest. I'll be upstairs opening mail."

Nancy slipped beneath the comforter and I slowly stroked her forehead. "They did too much." Seconds later, Nancy had entered dreamland.

I whispered, "I forgot to tell you that Joannie and Janis did the cleaning."

After quietly closing the bedroom door, I raced upstairs to our family room for a final check. Everything was ready. Each minute seemed like an hour. I tiptoed downstairs three times. A faint smile brushed Nancy's lips, but her eyes remained closed.

An eternity later, I heard a faint, "Winnie?" in the distance.

"I'm up here, Nancy. I've brought wine and snacks."

"I'll be right up."

When I heard Nancy at the bottom step, I jumped up to meet her mid stairway.

"Here, put this on." I placed a blue fleece ski hat on Nancy's head and pulled the front down just above the bottom of her nose so it covered her eyes. "No peeking. I have a small home-coming surprise for you."

"Winnie, what are you up to now?" Nancy shook her head but complied with my request. I led her up the last step and into the middle of our upstairs family room.

"Are you ready?" I asked her.

I slowly raised the stocking hat above Nancy's eyes. She blinked twice as she refocused her eyes and then her whole body flinched as if hit by a bolt of lightning. In front of her was an oak bookcase that spanned the entire far wall of our family room. Neatly arranged were all her favorite books, randomly spaced between the many knick-knacks I had collected from the hospital, past trips, and even some "coming home" gifts from friends.

Nancy quickly sat down on the couch. She hugged me as I whispered into her ear, "The shelves are adjustable for different sizes of books and whatever else you want on them. I just added a few things so you would have an idea of what's possible."

Nancy's head tilted to rest on my shoulder. "I love it, Winnie. You shouldn't have . . ."

With a start, Nancy's head lifted from its perch. "What happened to the TV?"

The giggle was mine this time.

"It's gone to TV retirement land."

Our family TV had once sat in front of the wall that now contained Nancy's bookcase. Once big and beautiful, it had finally surpassed twenty years in age. It was so old that when I watched a basketball game in its last years, the score was too fuzzy to read, and its colors were dull and faded.

"But what are we going to do?"

"Don't worry, my love. I know you'll be spending lots of time in this room over the next six months. When you're not reading, you can watch whatever your heart desires."

As I was speaking to Nancy, I slid the remote from my back pocket, pointed it at the bookcase, and pushed the button. A movie screen slowly descended from behind the fascia at the top of the bookcase. The screen was large—one hundred inches wide to be exact. I pushed another button. The huge screen filled with life-size faces and sound filled the room from in front of us, from each side, and behind us. Nancy turned around and discovered why she had been asked to wear a blindfold. New speakers and a projector hung from the ceiling behind her.

"Surround sound? It's the biggest TV I've ever seen!"

Nancy's eyes were not only wide—they were moist. I handed her a Kleenex and I took one for myself, too.

Nancy put her head on my shoulder again and closed her eyes. "Is it all right if I shut my eyes for a moment?"

"Yes, sweetheart. You rest. We can watch TV later. I plan on us being here a long time."

Summary: Home at last.

Thanks again,

Winnie

The Essence of Happiness

May 7, 6:16 a.m.

Dear Friends and Family,

My recent silence reflects a relatively tranquil five weeks. The past month has been more calming than a night at the symphony, balmier than a tropical beach at sunset, and gentler than a summer afternoon breeze.

After almost a year of turmoil, I am home with Nancy.

Though I've always tried to appreciate each and every day, I didn't fully realize that the most mundane things can be fun. I used to dread such tasks as doing the laundry, cleaning the house, or unpacking from a long trip away. Now every daily activity has joy attached because it is done with or for Nancy. And the things that I already cherished are even more special—a tasty meal prepared in our kitchen, movies and the NBA playoffs on our new home theatre, or walks in the woods along the river.

A week ago, as I examined three daffodils poking their bright-yellow heads through ground still covered by snow, I couldn't help but wonder about many things in my life.

Is Nancy as excited as I am to be far away from nurses and needles, sterile smells and scant scenery, bells and buzzers?

Is she enjoying our small, secluded island of paradise, savoring each moment like a sip of fine wine?

Is she still consumed with making it through each day?

Is she worrying about tomorrow?

And am I selfish to want her to be with me every moment of the day?

We've been at home now for five weeks, sleeping together in our comfortable bed. As always, I awaken first. I quietly linger to watch her gentle breathing, but since today is her weekly Salt Lake City doctor's appointment, I know Nancy has to get up two hours earlier than her normal 11 a.m. rising time.

As an alarm, I gently rub her head, which is covered increasingly with hair. It is no longer stubble standing straight in the air. The finely peppered strands are soft and long enough to twirl and run my fingers through gently. Slowly one eye, then the other, opens. The brilliance of their sky-blue color strikes me and momentarily brings heat to my face.

"Good morning, Nancy. How do you feel this morning?"

Nancy hesitates, wrinkling her forehead. She puts her hand on top of mine and rubs her head with me.

"It finally hit me last night, Winnie. I almost woke you up."

"What, my love?"

Nancy sits up and puts her hand on my right cheek while placing a kiss on the other.

"I'm happy. I am really happy."

Nancy's smile widens, reinforcing her words as I remove a Kleenex and feign wiping my nose.

Instead, I gently and delicately touch my eyes.

Summary: Nancy and I are at home, living almost normally. And we are both daring to be happy again.

All our love,

Winnie

A Toast to Regularity

May 22, 10:04 p.m.

Dear Friends and Family,

In my recurring fantasy, I want our home to be filled with nothing but wine and roses. I want each succeeding day to be better than the last. But in reality, all seven-month post-transplant patients face complications.

When Nancy has a "busy" day (going to the store, entertaining a guest, taking too long a walk), the next day she is often fatigued. Most of the time, the following day will be spent in bed—and if a bodily system changes even slightly, we brace ourselves.

At the six-week post-homecoming mark, Nancy experienced a major change. Over a three-day period, her GI tract became increasingly irritated. An emergency trip to the Blood and Marrow Transplant Clinic left my own stomach aggravated nearly as badly as Nancy's.

"Well, Nancy, we should have results back from your culture by tomorrow. If we don't find an infection, we'll have to consider the other possibility—graft-versus-host."

I masked a deep, audible sigh as I heard this unwelcome news. Things have been going so well for more than a full month. Yet in a heartbeat, we receive a reminder that we are still part of "transplant world." For us, each day is surely precious. But each day can also be fragile.

Nancy squeezed my hand, comforting me. I felt slightly embarrassed because she was the one with the IV fluids running into her vein. Her gesture did give me renewed strength, even resolve, to face the unwanted possibilities. But this time, the news was once again good.

"Nancy, now that we've filled up your tank, you can go home. But you need to drink, drink, and drink. If you get dehydrated again, we'll have to put you back in the hospital." Once again, Nancy took these words as a personal challenge. By the time we received a phone call the next day, there was a bottle of water or Gatorade on every table and night stand in the house.

"Nancy, this is Rene. We already have our answer—your stool culture grew C. difficile."

I have lost count of the number of GI germs Nancy has contracted, but this was a new one. C. difficile (Clostridium difficile, or C. diff) is a gastrointestinal bacterial infection that affects patients who have been on multiple antibiotics. Nancy's giant pillbox overflows with medicines that probably make such news inevitable. In fact, Rene said it was surprising she hadn't contracted C. diff earlier.

"We've requested a medicine called Flagyl at the pharmacy, Nancy. Remember, keep drinking. We want to see you back in the clinic in five days—unless you're having problems."

Nancy has continued to drink vigorously, though it is oftentimes a struggle.

Flagyl is a particularly foul medicine that leaves any patient taking it feeling nauseated because of its metallic taste. Nancy was not the exception. Even though she is currently on twenty-eight pills per day, she lamented, "I would rather take twice as many pills instead of swallowing one Flagyl, Winnie." She pinched her nose and forced down the first Flagyl pill of the day. She would have to swallow three more before bedtime. When I heard the retching sound of dry heaves, I raced to the kitchen to obtain a spoonful of peanut butter. (It is the best food we have discovered thus far to mask the horrible aftertaste of Flagyl.)

The next four days were not exactly fun, even though we were home at Woodland. When it was not raining, it was gray—inside and out. Nancy felt terrible, and her stomach discomfort and activity remained unchanged. Sleeping became her favorite activity, making the time pass and getting her to the next pill-taking session. On day five of the Flagyl regimen, we took another stool culture to Salt Lake City. By the end of the following day, the results were ready.

"Hello. This is Malinda from Bone Marrow. Nancy's culture is still positive for C. diff. She must have a resistant germ."

One of my top-ten fears has always been that Nancy might acquire a resistant germ. I gripped the phone tightly as I pondered the significance. I realized that Nancy can't exist with everything running like a broken faucet through her GI tract.

"We need to change medicines, Winnie. We're going to try Vancomycin."

(I know this drug well. Vancomycin, or Vanco as it is routinely called, is one of medicine's most powerful drugs. It is used in situations when all other antibiotics fail.)

"Thanks Malinda. Nancy is asleep, but I will leave her a note and run to the pharmacy immediately."

I hid my fears from Nancy, trying to be a husband and not her doctor. She was able to start the new medicine within the hour because I elected to obtain it in Park City, rather than the longer drive to the hospital pharmacy in Salt Lake City. Disappointingly, the day after we started the medicine, Nancy's bathroom trips increased and we had to return to the hospital for IV fluids and a repeat culture. Thankfully, Nancy was allowed to come home, but more of each passing day has been spent sleeping. I held my breath each time the phone rang. When another day dragged past, I knew the culture results had to be available. I couldn't wait any longer.

"Blood and Marrow Transplant Clinic. This is Marilyn."

Marilyn was the secretary of the Blood and Marrow Transplant Clinic. She was a kind, pleasant, grandmotherly woman—but she was new.

"Hi Marilyn, this is Nancy Winn's husband. I wondered if you could pull up Nancy's stool culture results on your computer. It's been two days and I believe the result should be ready."

"Certainly. Let's see. The C. diff. culture? Here it is. It looks like it's positive."

My heart sank like a boat's anchor. My eyes were moist. I had done some medical reading to see what happens if the Vanco didn't work. Shockingly, no other options were listed.

"Wait. I'm sorry, Winnie. That was the first culture, done on May 12. The one done two days ago on the twentieth is negative."

My heart returned to its proper anatomic position after tumbling over and over with joy.

"Thank you *so* much, Marilyn."

The Vanco had done its job. Nancy's C. diff., or "my bug" as she tells her friends, is gone for now. But deplorably, Nancy's stomach problems still persisted. So we visited the clinic the very next day to be certain we were on the correct course.

"I know it seems strange that with the C. diff. gone you are still having difficulty, Nancy. We need to wait until you finish the Vanco course to see if your bowel recovers. It's been through a lot."

I didn't verbalize or say what I was really thinking: *"Her whole body has been through a lot, Malinda."*

But we know how to wait.

If nothing else, leukemia has taught us patience.

The next day's brilliant sunshine lifted Nancy's mood. Even in her weakened state, we ventured outside to observe the many birds returning from their winter "homes away from home." As the distant mountains on the horizon slowly swallowed the sun, Nancy gripped her pillbox. She raised her glass as she took the last Vanco. "To the passing of 'my bug,'" she whispered while we clinked glasses filled with strawberry-flavored Gatorade.

Despite the world's most comfortable bed, my next two nights were restless. But by the third night, I was finally lost in dreamland and Nancy was again eating, walking, and most importantly, visiting the bathroom less regularly.

Summary: Nancy had yet another setback, but she is once again back on track.

Our very best,

Winnie

A Very Important Anniversary

May 29, 11:09 p.m.

Dear Friends and Family,

Over the past many months of illness and uncertainty, Nancy's disease has given us many new dates to celebrate.

Her new transplant birthday.

The one-hundred-day post-transplant milestone.

Our joyous return home.

Each and every negative bone marrow test.

Tonight, however, when I looked at the time and date—I didn't know whether to celebrate or cry.

Last year on this date and at this time, give or take several minutes, the emergency room doctor at LDS Hospital confirmed my fear that Nancy had leukemia. Tonight, Nancy has made it to her "one year out" tests and she has passed all her tests with flying colors. A year out, there is still no sign or hint of leukemia recurrence. Her new, infant bone marrow is maturing nicely. And her lungs are working just fine, recovering from the damage caused by the many toxic drugs.

Despite the bumps, the overall picture is crystal clear: Nancy is remarkably better than two months ago and light years different from this day one year ago.

Summary: Last May 29, I was told Nancy had leukemia. The cancer doctor told me he doubted Nancy would survive the holiday weekend. I have not forgotten that fateful night even though a full year has passed. I feel blessed and in awe. And I want you all to know something else that is very important, too—we couldn't have made it without your support.

Warmly,

Winnie

Hope instead of Uncertainty

July 9, 2:38 a.m.

Dear Friends and Family,

I didn't plan to write much until this coming October when Nancy would celebrate her one-year transplant anniversary—her new transplant birthday. However, yesterday (July 8) was another significant day that I almost unwittingly forgot—Nancy's other birthday (her fifty-eighth).

Nancy was able to fully enjoy her "birthdate" compared to last year when she'd arrived home just after the first round of chemotherapy treatments.

On this birthdate, Nancy was able to eat a small salad and take several bites of one of her favorite foods, a rib eye steak.

On this birthdate, Nancy took three bites of carrot cake saturated with scoops of vanilla ice cream sitting beside it.

On this birthdate, instead of nasal oxygen and a central IV line for drugs, Nancy had a pillbox next to her plate, whose contents are steadily decreasing (down to twenty-two pills per day).

On this birthdate, instead of celebrating like it may be her last, Nancy drank wine and toasted to many more.

On this birthdate, Nancy knows that if things continue like the last two months, subsequent birthdays will be filled with warmth, happiness, and even fun.

Best of all, on this birthdate, Nancy's smile is confident and without pain. There is abundant hope instead of abundant uncertainty.

Summary: On Nancy's fifty-eighth "birthdate" yesterday, we had a true and utterly complete celebration.

Our very best,

Winnie

Such a Long, Long Way

July 17, 11:17 p.m.

Dear Friends and Family,

When Nancy awoke this morning, she announced, "I was dreaming you were making me a peanut butter and jelly sandwich, Winnie."

"Now there's a dream that could come true. Do you want one?"

"Actually, I'm not hungry. Maybe in a little while."

A little while passed, so I asked, "What would you think about a peanut butter surprise, Nancy? I can add mayonnaise and bananas instead of jelly. I can make it just the way you like your sandwich."

"I don't think so. What I really crave is canned peas—over rice."

Nancy and I share many "favorite" foods.

Anchovies.

Popcorn.

Strawberry preserves on "normal" PB+J's.

Peas?

Peas never ever grace my plate. Just give me a PB+J any time—even with grape jelly. But Nancy has strange cravings while her new immunity is "setting up shop." She is slowly eating more things, and more of the things that she does eat. Nearly every day, she eats one full meal, along with strange snacks for which she has a craving. She has returned to her pre-illness weight, which is a good thing.

"Peas?"

I look to the back of a bottom kitchen shelf where a Green Giant smiles back at me and obediently respond, "Let me see what I can do."

My schedule is varied, so weekends often find me at the office. But during this particular spring and summer, with Jayna living in Salt Lake City where she is finishing her last semester of college, Saturdays and Sundays usually mean a visit from our daughter. Consequently, for the first time in recent memory, weekends are distinct from other days of the week.

We try to have at least one complete meal at the dining room table.

We always watch a rented movie in our new home theater.

We even enjoy a cocktail or glass of wine if Nancy's ever-changing taste buds are willing.

"To you, Mom. I love you," Jayna toasts on this summer Saturday in July.

"Why always to me, Jayna? Is it just because I'm still standing?"

Laughter emanates from all four corners of our table—even Jaret laughs while sipping sparkling cider.

"Yes, Mom. You've been through so much this year."

"You know, I've been thinking. It really wasn't that bad. And there are days now that I feel healthy—almost normal."

Both Jayna and I simply roll our eyes and shake our heads.

Summary: We really appreciate your many thoughts and prayers. Though you don't (and won't) hear from me as often now, unlike Nancy, I do remember—the frightening times, the bad times, and how your support helped each member of our family. What a long, long way we've come.

Sincerely,

Winnie

A Great Day for a Haircut

October 27, 4:44 p.m.

Dear Friends and Family,

The light streaming through the window is a little less intense in our corner of the world now; our lawn is hiding beneath a shallow blanket of brilliant gold aspen leaves sprinkled with an early season snowfall.

I realize that it's been several months since my last update, but life has been terrifically unexciting. Summer and fall have been filled with bright sunshine, both inside and outside our Woodland retreat. Nancy continues to slowly recuperate, experiencing more good days than bad. In general, our family, and Nancy in particular, has savored each and every day without hospital food.

So why write now?

Today is October 27.

On our family's revised post-illness calendar, October 27 is our biggest holiday. On this day last year, Nancy received her gift—the transplant.

Today is our day to reflect and be grateful. It is the day we are finally allowed by the National Marrow Donor Program to initiate the process that may lead to our finding out the identity of Nancy's donor. Each member of the Winn family would like the opportunity to personally thank Nancy's donor.

While Nancy went to Park City to obtain the ingredients for our celebratory dinner, I filled out the proper transplant registry paperwork and posted it in our mailbox with great satisfaction. I can think of nothing more gratifying than to shake our donor's hand and have him meet Nancy's many friends and supporters. If we are able to contact him and he consents, we plan to fly him to Park City for a big party in his honor. We'd like him to meet as many of you as possible.

When Nancy returned home in the early afternoon, I inquired, "Hi, Nancy. How was Park City?" My bride gave me a look we exchange frequently. "What do you think?" dangled from the corners of her lips. She won't ask. It's part of a game we both enjoy—which of us will break first?

"It was fun, Winnie. I ran into Jane at the Albertson's and Susan at Linens N Things. Both asked about you. And I found a razor for Jaret."

(Nancy finally has enough strength to make local shopping trips, and her taste buds have finally recovered. Much to my delight, she is also cooking again.)

"Can I have a sip, Nancy? I'm dying of thirst."

Nancy picks up the sixteen-ounce Coke cup sitting between the driver and passenger seats. "Sure, Winnie," she said as she handed me the half-empty drink. After taking a big gulp, I spit the contents almost across the driveway. "What is that?"

Between fits of laughter, Nancy replies, "Just one of my 'combos'—I start with Mountain Dew, combine it with lemonade, and then add vanilla Coke. Oh, and raspberry tea at the very end. I forgot—you don't like tea."

I surrounded her with my arms. "You really got me. You haven't made one of your 'combinations' in a very long time. It must be a special day." Then, softly rubbing her head with the back of one hand, I could no longer ignore Nancy's now beautiful hair. "I like your hair. Do you?"

Nancy shook her head from side to side, pleased with her pyric victory. I had commented first. "Yep, I do. I wondered if you'd notice or at least would say something."

I twisted her new curls between my thumb and index finger. Over just an hour or so ago, those curls hung two or three inches longer. It was her first haircut in seventeen months. Bald, long, or (now) short, she always looks great.

Nancy was diagnosed with AML on May 29. After achieving the first remission, we were told she had, at best, a 5%–10% chance of survival. With the transplant, her chance of survival increased to 50%. And by a hundred days post-transplant, we heard incredibly good news from her doctor: "Nancy, you made it through an extremely rough procedure. By making it this far, you have an 80% chance of a cure."

On this day last year, less than two ounces of bone marrow stem cells flowed into Nancy's vein. And the news from Nancy's doctor today when he called with results was the most wonderful news that a person can receive.

"Nancy's one year (post-transplant) bone marrow shows no sign of leukemia. The donor stem cells are healthy. A recurrence of leukemia will get more and more unlikely as the months pass. By two years, Nancy's risk will be less than 5%."

Our next challenge?

We will need to get Nancy off the remaining bone marrow–suppressing medicines so she can be around larger groups and travel again. Right now, heading into the winter flu season, she still is at greater risk (than you or I) for normal and unusual infections. Since her new immune system is literally in its infancy, Nancy has to redo her "baby" shots such as polio and tetanus in the next six months once she tapers the medicine that has been suppressing it.

And after that, the next big milestone according to Dr. Pulsipher?

"Once Nancy is off her immune-suppressing medicines and makes it another three months, have a big party. At that point, it'll be highly unlikely her graft will attack her organs. And she will be able to resume a more normal life without much worry about germs."

You may not hear from me until close to the three month's post-medicine day, but I can promise each of you that you will be invited to the big party.

Summary: On her "new" birthday, Nancy had her first haircut in almost a year and a half. We also heard the sweetest of results from her recent testing. There is no leukemia in Nancy's body. Simply put, her doctors couldn't have been more pleased with her progress. Nor could we.

My very best,

Winnie

Growing Up Is Hard

October 31, 10:35 p.m.

Dear Friends and Family,

When in rapid succession this morning Nancy answered the phone with the smile reserved for first Jayna and then Jaret, I decided it might be a good time to update you on the kids—especially since she related to me everything she heard on the other end.

"Hi, Mom. Guess what? I just gave blood."

"That's wonderful, Jaret. You might help save a life."

"That's what I'm hoping for."

I know I mentioned in one of my very early letters that when Jaret was in kindergarten, he disliked everything about Halloween. "I don't want a costume," he'd protest on the day most kids couldn't wait for school to show off their newest outfit. Not only did he hate costumes, he was afraid of masks, and Jaret even despised carved pumpkins. As he grew up, so did his "blacklist." It expanded to all things medical. He would hide when we passed graveyards. He had an aversion to bones and blood, until his mother got sick.

Jaret stepped up big time when his mom became ill. He spent more time in the hospital last year than most kids do in their entire lives. He even relieved Jayna for a few of the all-night shifts with Nancy. And I can't forget his efforts to clean up the bloody mess when Nancy inadvertently pulled her central IV line out in the Salt Lake City apartment kitchen. So it is only fitting that Jaret has matured enough to donate blood as he finishes his last semester of college—voluntarily.

As far as Jayna's status, yesterday, I received a call at 7:45 a.m.

"Hi Daddy, did I wake you?"

"No, Jayna, I'm the first shift today. I'm on my way to work."

"I am, too. This is hard, Dadder. It's so early. I'm used to getting ten hours of sleep a night. Today that would have meant getting up around twelve. I guess I'll have to call it a night a bit earlier than two in the morning. We went dancing last night."

"I have a better idea, Jayna. Why don't you just tell everyone that you speak Spanish and need a midday siesta? We really don't want work interfering with your dancing."

"You're absolutely no help, Dadder. Well, I'm here. So have a great day. I love you."

Jayna graduated college this summer and began her first job while she (like many of her peers) is figuring out what to do next. Five days each week, she sits at a desk working as an online travel agent for Overstock.com in Salt Lake City. It's great having her nearby Nancy and me. And on some mornings, it's worth a few good laughs as she adjusts to the "working" world that the rest of us live in every day.

Summary: The fog of the past year is slowly lifting for our children. It is so wonderful to see them returning to ordinary lives. Nancy and I feel the same way.

With much love,

Winnie

Christmas in April

April 4, 2:13 a.m.

Dear Friends and Family,

April in the mountains heralds the final gasp of winter. The ski resorts close. The once dominant all-white covering fades from the landscape. By the time errant snow patches hide only under trees or on tops of faraway peaks, I pretend the holidays aren't that long ago. I remove the Christmas cards I received in December from a special drawer in my desk. Most years, the mountains are completely green by the time I start my yearly epistle. So by my timeline, the fact that you are receiving my "Holiday Greetings" in April is really early this year.

Why?

Milestones.

In my lifetime, I can't remember another year when our family celebrated more momentous events. And none was bigger than this past week on April 2. Two days ago, Nancy swallowed her final Cyclosporine tablet. (Cyclosporine is the medicine designed to hold her donor graft immunity in check. It is the medicine that has kept her away from crowds and out of airplanes.)

As Nancy swallowed that last pill, I reminded her, "Three months from now, we can travel anywhere our hearts desire. Where do you want to go first?"

Barring any setbacks, Nancy will have no restrictions. By then, the twenty other pills per day should be down to just vitamins and a few medicines unrelated to leukemia. She should also be well on her way to redoing her "baby" immunizations.

What am I trying to convey?

On Christmas Day three and a half months ago, Nancy resided in the hospital. She was beautifully bald and in the middle of her treatment. She had been in and out of the hospital multiple times, both for treatments and for complications from those treatments. Many days I worried about what came next. On other days, Nancy was so sick I wondered if she would make it to the following day. Good times were measured in minutes and hours, and, on rare occasions, full days.

Now Nancy is home in her own bed. She has a full head of hair that even requires haircuts. Good times are now measured in weeks and, soon, months. Consequently, for our family this year, I've declared April 2 as Christmas Day. I am sending our "Holiday Greetings" out today not only to those on my update list but also to those on my Christmas list.

With Nancy taking the last pill (Cyclosporine) that has been holding her immune system in check, her transplant will gain full strength sometime during the next ninety days. She will finally obtain the "protection" she needs against germs that will allow her to return to a completely normal life. We have been excitedly waiting for this day. It is a great and wonderful reason to celebrate Christmas.

Though Nancy's milestone obviously surpasses everything else, a few other high points are worth mentioning in the same way I have traditionally undertaken my annual review for the last twenty or so years.

All right, I'll get mine over with first.

Every year, our partnership has donated a scholarship to a graduating senior of the Park City High School interested in a medical field. In 1990, the recipient was Charlie Morrison. He excelled in college and went on to medical school—which made it especially gratifying when he joined our partnership in 2004. Not only is Charlie a gifted and caring physician, he is an easily loved human bursting with a good sense of humor. We've become fast friends.

Last fall Charlie and I were talking about medicine, mountain biking, and family when he told me his father was about to retire. "How old is your dad?" I inquired. "Almost sixty," he replied in a tone that made sixty sound like it was just short of the century mark. When I related my conversation later that night to Nancy, she hooted as loudly as me. She recognized the irony—I am due to turn the big "6-0" in February, just like his father.

The day after our conversation, Charlie and I climbed for more than an hour to reach the top of a lengthy and sometimes steep mountain trail. I reached the summit long before Charlie. I didn't tell him I was a few days older than his dad. The mountain bike ride was a personal milestone, if not outright challenge, given Charlie's words about age.

The kids' landmarks easily dwarf mine.

"Hi, Jayna. Guess what came in the mail today? Are you even a little excited?"

"Oh, well. I guess a tiny bit. Is it pretty, Dadder?"

When Jayna rushed home after her junior year abroad in Peru to be with (and help) her mother, she transferred from Vassar College to the University of Utah. Nancy and I were heartsick that she would not spend her senior year with her friends and classmates, taking the best upper-level courses while participating in the many traditional things seniors do at a small college. But Jayna was adamant. "I want to be here with you, Mommy. I want to help you fight your battle along with Dad."

Jayna's final year was different from her other college senior friends. She took basic courses in international studies because Utah didn't have the same upper-level courses available at Vassar in her Latin American Studies major. Nights were spent in the hospital alternating sleepovers with me, not in the dorms or clubs being young and carefree with friends. Her thoughts were dominated by her mother's lab values and medicines rather than daydreams about dates or planning for graduate school. At year's end, she chose not to "walk" for graduation, opting instead to wait for her diploma to come in the mail.

Still, as I pulled Jayna's diploma from the University of Utah envelope that had just been delivered to our mailbox, I was nearly overcome with emotion. "It's not pretty, Jayna. It's beautiful—just like you."

"Oh, Dadder. You're such a soft touch." Even over the phone, Jayna could see my face from hearing my voice.

"But, Dadder. For the last time—I have no regrets. It was worth it."

Jayna is now a college graduate. Despite having a GPA that would allow her to do pretty much anything (4.0 at the University of Utah and 3.9 at Vassar), her next step will be having fun after a difficult twenty-two months. She has decided to remain nearby for at least another year, so she has found a job in Salt Lake City and, for the very first time, her very own apartment. We see her often, and she continues to be exceptionally close with her mother.

And Jaret?

When Nancy came home from the hospital at the end of last March, she was light years better than the many months when she would fall asleep in the middle of a meal. Still it was not uncommon for her to have far fewer waking hours than those spent sleeping and napping. But her decreased strength could not dampen her singular purpose—to help Jaret through his final days of college. By his last semester, the task seemed formidable even to Nancy. His ending class was titled "Research Methods." And what did that entail? Numerous presentations, a twenty-page paper, and the design of a project.

Many nights, Nancy would confide, "C minus is all he needs, Winnie. But I don't know if it's possible." Speaking in front of groups and writing long papers are nearly impossible tasks for someone with autism, like Jaret. But he had made it almost to the end and even had a 3.4 GPA. So with Nancy's usual unwavering support and constant help, Jaret made an A minus. He will receive his diploma in June. Quite honestly, we never would have predicted such an accomplishment. There are now two new college graduates in our family.

A final story about Nancy's journey and how far we've come.

I am the luckiest guy in the world. The other day, I had two dates to the afternoon matinee, the kind of movie Nancy is allowed to attend since there are few other people in the audience. In fact, the three of us were the only ones in the entire old-fashioned movie house in the nearby hamlet of Kamas. We could talk normally, laugh as loud as we wanted, and throw popcorn (not that we did) with impunity. On the way home,

I was designated chauffeur, since Nancy and our good friend Joan decided to sit in the back seat. It was totally appropriate, since they ignored me and did all the chatting, like two school-girls at a sleepover. Nancy was her old self. I heard frequent giggles in the midst of conversations ranging from haircuts to world politics.

One particular part of their chat caught my attention like no other conversation in the last year and a half as Joan related that a common friend was about to undergo chemotherapy for breast cancer. After sharing the sad moment, Nancy responded, "I'd be happy to talk to her if you think it would help. I could tell her what it was like when I had leukemia."

I almost ran off the road. In my rearview mirror, Joan nodded her head while giving me a wink when she saw me looking at her with raised eyebrows and a surprised but totally pleased look on my face. At long last, my bride was ready to put her illness behind her once and for all.

Nancy is not alone. Our whole family looks forward to an even more ordinary life. But we won't ever forget the many kindnesses of so many during our long and difficult ordeal.

So at a time that I have designated Christmas for us—I'll be thinking of you often.

Summary: I declared Christmas for our family this year on another landmark day. And I am thrilled to declare that Nancy continues her path toward normalcy.

All our love,

Winnie

Transplant + Two

October 20, 10:11 p.m.

Dear Friends and Family,

Do you remember this?

"If Nancy makes it two years beyond her transplant, have a party. A BIG PARTY."

I do—as clear today as when it was said nearly a year ago.

Nancy's transplant doctor made this statement in response to my question, "When can we feel comfortable Nancy has beaten her disease?"

Actually, I doubt you remember my October 27 update on her one-year transplant "birthday." In fact, I doubt you distinctly remember many of my past updates, since it has been over six months since I last communicated with you. As with many of you, I went silent once Nancy "got well" for a purpose. I hoped to save my final update to invite you to the BIG PARTY.

As a matter of fact, Nancy's two-year post-transplant anniversary is next week—October 27. I had planned to use this final communiqué as the invitation to the BIG PARTY where we would offer our heartfelt thanks to everyone who helped these past few years. Instead, Nancy will be in Georgia, visiting her family and friends. So I won't even be at the small party that will be occurring several thousand miles away. (I guess somebody has to work.) Nonetheless I hope, like me, that you'll take a moment to smile or a make toast (or both) at the thought of Nancy reaching the noteworthy two-year mark. And I hope you know that both she and I will be thinking of you because we are forever grateful. Two years is a very long time, and you have been with us the entire way.

So, what is life like now that we have reached our final milestone?

It is still early in the evening, but Nancy sits beside me, already in dreamland. A gentle grin is splashed across her lips. It has been like this hundreds of times during our thirty years together. Me, in the dimming light, looking past her through the tiny oval window, trying to decipher what images I can make out of clouds that too swiftly pass by us. I often wonder what images are playing in her mind's theatre as she peacefully sleeps on my shoulder. But this time is more noteworthy than any of the previous occasions.

Yes, we've reached our cruising altitude of 39,000 feet.

Yes, the seatbelt sign has gone off, and I feel just a touch safer.

Yes, I savor the freedom of feeling no phones or distractions.

We are finally airborne and I delight in the anticipation of being "on our way."

Instead of laughing quietly to myself at how quickly Nancy has fallen asleep, I am overwhelmed with emotion and fight my likely tears. Two years and five months ago, it was beyond my wildest dreams that Nancy would ever again be healthy enough to travel—actually, that she would even still be with me.

So where did Nancy choose for her first big trip after her battle with death?

Chicago.

Chicago, you say?

I know Chicago has famous deep-dish pizza and an adored (though highly unsuccessful) baseball team, but Nancy doesn't even like baseball. Worse yet, Chicago's basketball team robbed our Utah Jazz of an NBA Championship not once, but twice.

So why then are we not heading to an exotic Caribbean beach or a mysterious African safari?

"Dad, guess what? I'm moving to Chicago. You know how I'm an English geek and how I love to read. I found an editing program at the University of Chicago that accepts college graduates and only takes one year to get a master's degree. What do you think?"

"I think it's great," I whisper into the telephone. *I don't tell Jayna that there are tears in my eyes and that they are not from sadness. Though I will miss you my dear Jayna, I am so happy you feel good enough about your mother's health to move forward. You donated two years of your life to assist me with Mom. But then again, you are like her. How can I thank you?* The words are silent, in my head.

Much has taken place in the two months since my conversation took place with Jayna. She is already living in her own apartment in Lincoln Park (Chicago), working as a search analyst at a Google company, and poised to start her night classes. And today, Jayna is preparing for her first visit from her mother and me. Significantly, the trip to Chicago will be our first trip together since Nancy's illness. (Today is also filled with joy because Jayna, like her mom, is finally recovering.)

Although my life has emerged from a pitch-black dark cave into almost blinding sunshine, there is still an occasional cloud. A few weeks ago, Nancy was enjoying the mundane, taking her car in for an oil change. For her, every trip is still an adventure, every small detail still an extra opportunity for an encounter. She and Jaret had dropped off the car and headed to a nearby shopping area on foot. They were distracted by a distinctive sports car, and while discussing its color and examining its shape, Nancy tripped and fell.

The result?

Forty minutes later, Nancy was in our office getting two broken fingers splinted. Selflessly, Jaret took me aside. "Dad, will Mom's broken fingers cause graft-versus-host disease?"

During Nancy's illness Jaret was often the forgotten one. Not verbal like his sister, during the really tough times when I only left the hospital for my work shifts, my face-to-face interactions with my son were few. He was in college finishing his last year and not often at home. Although he did spend several "hospital" nights with Nancy along the way, he wasn't in the regular rotation with Jayna and me. Still it was clear he had the same worries, the same ups and downs, and now, the same scars. When Nancy sneezes, isn't as hungry as usual, looks tired, or, in this case, falls, Jaret (like Jayna and me) immediately become concerned and think the worst.

In reality, it will be a very long time before the despair, concern, and grief of our past nightmares totally subside. But we are making positive, albeit slow, progress.

"No, Jaret. Breaking a bone should have no effect on Mom's immune system. Normal people break bones all the time and they heal quickly."

Jaret, his finest smile easing the tightness from his brow, replies, "I didn't think so, Dad. I just wanted to be sure."

Summary: Nancy recovery's is going well. It has been nearly two years since Nancy's transplant and the news continues to be favorable.

With love,

Winnie

Castles by the Sea

October 31, 2:34 a.m.

Dear Friends and Family,

Nancy took another airplane trip this past summer after being told she could travel and be around people. The destination was Marblehead, Massachusetts, for the wedding of Stefanie Freeman, the daughter of her good friend Lyn. We've known Stefanie since birth. Nancy was allowed to attend this joyous event, her goal for the entire last year, because she now has an immune system that should protect her from normal germs. The experience exceeded all our expectations. She visited with old friends, drank and ate the best of Boston, and danced as much (or more) than even the youngest of the wedding guests. The next day, I returned to Utah for work while Nancy stayed an extra day with our friends John and Cheryl Jermyn.

John asked Nancy what she wanted to do, and in Nancy's low-key, never-a-burden style, she replied, "Maybe we could go to the ocean." In less than thirty minutes, Nancy was retrieving bucket after bucket of sand and mud to help John's kids, Cole and Jaclyn, construct a sand castle. When the moat surrounding their intricate multilevel castle was completed, John dashed into the ocean to wash off the sand. Unfortunately, he found the water only slightly warmer than the Arctic Ocean, so he quickly retreated. Nancy, on the other hand, slowly waded in. First, up to her ankles, then up to her waist, and finally up to her neck. She floated and splashed and even fully submerged her hair-covered head. For nearly an hour, she frolicked like a three-year-old in a wading pool. Later, finally dry and sitting on her towel at the water's edge, she gazed at the horizon, the expression on her face almost as far away.

Nancy grew up spending entire days at the beaches of Georgia and Florida, and her fondest childhood memories are intertwined with sand and sea. She turned to John, and though I was not there, John didn't have to describe the look on her face when he recounted what she softly told him: *"I never thought I'd get to do this again."* John became as choked up then as I am now as I share Nancy's proclamation with each of you, my dear friends.

The truth is that Nancy has experienced imminently facing one's mortality and then getting a second chance. In reality, her journey hasn't made her more loving, more caring, or more wonderful than before. But she is more aware.

And me?

I am almost speechless.

How do I describe where we are today?

Glorious and magnificent are probably close depictions, with a splash of humbleness for Nancy having made me more aware, too.

Have I changed?

My friend Fred says I press the "easy" button more often than in the past because I don't sweat the small stuff as I once did. But as I sit here and reflect, I realize my biggest change is how I feel. Good, caring people still exist in this world. And Nancy and I have heard from and met more than our fair share of these people during her extended illness.

We thank you once again for your many kind thoughts, words, and actions. We are forever in your collective debt for helping to get us through the hard times.

Summary: *Nancy is "out of the woods" and leukemia-free.*

> With all our love and all
> our thankfulness—always,
>
> Winnie

Conclusion

For me, Yellowstone National Park is like no other place on earth. It is where Nancy walked into my life. It is where Nancy and I lived for two full summers during the early years of our relationship. It is the place where our children developed their love for nature. The park is where Nancy and I learned to hike and backpack. We learned, as we explored its countless trails, about flowers and trees and the interrelatedness of an ecosystem. And, most important, Yellowstone is not only where we fell in love with the outdoors and where we came to love solitude but also where we fell deeply in love.

In many ways, we grew up in Yellowstone. As Nancy and I became the people that we are today, so too did we grow and evolve. We grew together. First, as a young man and woman, then as a fledgling couple, and then, not so many years later, as husband and wife. For these reasons, Nancy and I decided to celebrate the five-year anniversary of her cancer-free recovery in the familiar, intensely meaningful, and comfortable surroundings of the park. We wanted to return to our roots. Our homecoming was a natural and very personal way for us to return to where our lives together began so many years ago.

Even today, I remember our triumphant return as if it were only yesterday. All I have to do is close my eyes and wave after wave of images, sights and sounds, and corresponding emotions take me back in time. Like the rhythmic and relentless beating of a drum, I am almost overwhelmed by the vividness and immediacy of these memories. I close my eyes and instantly I can once again see Nancy reading every word on the front and back covers of the familiar maps, edges worn from repeated unfolding and refolding, before carefully opening the map of Yellowstone fully on her lap.

"Same old map, Winnie," she declares. "Nothing's changed."

"What's your fancy?" I inquire while dropping my right arm from the steering wheel and brushing Nancy's left cheek with the back of my hand. A quick glance reveals a crescendo of sentiment across Nancy's face.

"I want our first stop to be Black Sand Basin."

Black Sand Basin, a name derived from the coarse, black gravel covering much of the area that had its origin in Obsidian volcanic glass, is a small part of the massive Upper Geyser Basin best known for the Old Faithful Geyser. Located on the opposite side of the major road leading into the Old Faithful Geyser Basin Area, it is usually not crowded with people like most geyser basins. Even better, the parking lot is most often empty.

About fifteen years into our thirty-year-plus marriage, Nancy declared the basin her favorite area in the park. At the time, it was close to our living quarters and a great place to take the kids when they were young. Not only did it contain a wide range of thermal features, it had benches for relaxing in relative privacy. As an added benefit, the scenery and atmosphere encourages reflection and contemplation. For Nancy, it has always been a hidden jewel.

After parking the car and proceeding on the boardwalk along Iron Spring Creek, we feel the wind in our faces and smell the not-unexpected sulfur odor of a geyser basin. "Funny," Nancy says as she grabs my hand, "I can remember being repulsed by that fragrance the first year. Now it smells almost good to me."

I look at Nancy and sense the enveloping warmth of her presence. She glows from head to toe.

"This is so amazing, Winnie. I thought of this moment so often when I was in the hospital. It was dreamlike then. I doubted I would return."

I am stunned by Nancy's admission. (But I am not prepared to admit that there were pain-filled days and sleepless nights when I thought we would not return together either.)

"Look!" she points out. "Right on cue."

Cliff Geyser, on the opposite edge of the creek, begins erupting as it does every few minutes all day long. After a strong eruption, about twenty feet high, the spray, like the sulfur smell, drifts our way in a mist that cools our faces. Nancy places a wet sulfuric kiss on my cheek and squeezes my hand.

As we stroll further, we observe dense steam rising from Sunset Lake. A massive thermal feature about sixty yards long and fifty yards wide, the lake's light-blue color is ringed with yellow and orange from the algae growing along its edges. During most of our prior visits, all we could see was the steam. Not today, because the same strong gust of wind that almost blew my Mountain Trails Foundation baseball cap off my head carries the steam away from the lake's surface, revealing the whole lake. Nancy revels at our good fortune with the giggle that I so dearly love, and then she tugs on my hand to let me know it is time to go.

At twenty-eight feet by fifty-five feet, Opalescent Pool is long and skinny. It is cooler than Black Sand Basin because its water is the runoff from the adjacent Spouter Geyser. Its opaque, medium-blue center is surrounded by deep brown on its periphery, revealing the bacteria that grow at the cooler temperature. What makes Opalescent Pool so extraordinary isn't the pool itself but rather the trees in and around it. When the pool first formed, the hot chemicals in the water killed the lodgepole pines. Over time, the repeated rising and falling water from the geyser that feeds the pool deposited white silica to the depth of several feet at the base of each of the trees. In case I had forgotten, Nancy reminds me, "I just love those bobby sock–looking trees."

Our next stop is Rainbow Pool, appropriately named because the entire rounded perimeter flashes and flaunts the colors of a bright rainbow. At one hundred feet across, its sky-blue middle is as clear as glass, and when I look into its depth, I can't see the bottom. The gentle surface bubbles remind me that it is a very warm pool and to not get too close to the boardwalk's threshold. Nancy squeezes my hand again and murmurs, "Isn't it incredibly beautiful?" I know how she feels. And before we move on, she whispers in my ear, "It is *soooo* good to be back."

At the end of the boardwalk is a bench overlooking the dark-green pool designated by the park service as Emerald Pool.

Though only a bit larger than a backyard swimming pool, it is one of the park's most well-known hot springs because its brilliant green color is different from the other pools in Yellowstone that sport varying shades of blue in their hearts. The green of Emerald Pool is even more distinctive because it is ringed by pale blue and bright orange.

Nancy and I sit on the bench at the edge of Emerald Pool, and after a minute, she lightly rests her head on my shoulder. In the distance, a red-tailed hawk circles high above the trees on the fringe of the thermal area. I sit silently and am totally fulfilled. Finally we are far, far away from the frightening nightmare of Nancy's illness.

Before I can ask Nancy about where we should go next, she lifts her head and engages me with eyes as blue as Rainbow Pool. She pulls off her left shoe and slips off her sock like she did in January over five years ago. Extending her leg beyond the ground-level boardwalk, she ever so lightly touches her big toe to a lonely clump of grass that somehow has managed to survive even though it is completely surrounded by the black sands only a few feet away from the blistering pool. Nancy puts an index finger to her lips cautioning me not to speak.

No worries, my love, I reflect silently.

You made it through, you survived, and you are well.

Together we have made it back home.

Finale

When the snowplows finally clear the highways leading into Yellowstone at the end of May, the all-too-brief period during which visitors can marvel at the splendor of the world's first National Park begins. Each year three and a half million sightseers tour the nearly five hundred miles of twisting two-lane roads before snow once again closes the park at the end of October. And every year during this five-month window, year in and year out, perfect memories can be experienced and captured for a lifetime.

On any given day, visitors from all over the world witness hundreds upon hundreds of bison from the nation's largest herd as they graze in the vast meadows in the southeast section of the park called the Hayden Valley. (Yellowstone is the only place in the United States where these shaggy beasts have lived continuously since prehistoric times.) Vacationers and park sightseers alike encounter both male and female Shiras moose feeding knee-deep in the pristine wetlands. And if they are lucky (as thousands are each year), a grizzly bear sighting can take place or even a fleeting glimpse of one of the recently reintroduced wild gray wolves frolicking with the members of its pack. The pronghorn antelope, the fastest land animal in North America, may even be observed running through the sagebrush at sixty miles an hour thereby exceeding the posted forty-five miles per hour maximum speed allowed on the park's roads.

I well remember the first time I visited Yellowstone. (It was many years ago and long before I met Nancy.) I encountered a tangle of cars blocking both lanes in the northeast section of the park, just outside of Mammoth, Wyoming. Getting out of my car like everyone else, I viewed a bighorn sheep perched in the notch of a formation of jagged rocks jutting above the road. Balanced like a king on his throne, the bighorn's grandeur was overwhelming. His eyes flashed like a shooting star, and I felt as if he was looking at me alone. He had eyes only for me. When he made a slow head motion resembling a nod before trotting down the far side of the rocks and out of sight, I knew deep inside me that I had discovered something that was both extraordinary and wondrous.

Later on during that very first early summer day in Yellowstone, I climbed up the gravel road to the summit and fire lookout of the 10,243-foot Mount Washburn. Near the top, I encountered a family of mountain goats, including two cute little twin kids with tiny white beards snuggling close to the furry warm body of their mother. Once again, I was utterly and totally enthralled.

Over the years, in addition to the larger animals that freely roam Yellowstone, I learned that almost everywhere in the park there are wild birds, including elegant great blue herons, magnificent trumpeter swans, sleek snowy egrets, and of course, magnificent bald and golden eagles. Common ravens and American crows join visitors in the campgrounds and picnic spots, along with least chipmunks and Uintah ground squirrels, all anxious for snacks from accommodating humans. Even though park rules discourage the feeding of animals, many do so anyway.

Memories of a solitary American white pelican with a cutthroat trout in his bill or two elk rutting to gain dominance in their herd during mating season have left an indelible and lifelong impression to this day. And I remember as if it were only yesterday once stopping to watch a one-ton bison scratch its back by dropping to the ground and rolling in the roadside sand directly to the right of my Subaru on a glorious, sunlit afternoon.

On that very first day so many years ago, by the time I had navigated nearly half the park, I fully awakened to the realization that I would never again wander very far from a place as hallowed as Yellowstone. (I have returned to Yellowstone almost annually from my home in Park City to rediscover the park's natural beauty and wildlife that has for many years comforted me during difficult times.)

Often, I recall being mesmerized by Tower Falls, a 132-foot waterfall that plunges in a perfect column of water and splashes onto the rocks at its base in a triumphant deep roar heard loudly from the lookout hundreds of feet away. As one of the park's largest of the 290 waterfalls that drop greater than fifteen feet, I remember once being momentarily frozen in reverence, time suspended as I watched the torrent flow powerfully downward amid the eroded rock pinnacles that frame the waterfall's entire length. It was only when a young Belgian couple asked if I would mind taking their picture that I snapped back to the present. The couple smiled shyly when they explained they were on their honeymoon.

Rivers, small ponds, and lakes sitting below peaks as high as 11,358 feet are omnipresent, and these bodies of water amid the overlooking mountains provide a striking backdrop for Yellowstone Lake, the water jewel of the park. Its 130-square-mile surface area of deep, crystal-clear blue water can be enjoyed from the many overlooks along the road that snakes around its northern border.

Sitting above 7,000 feet in elevation, Lake Yellowstone is the country's largest high-elevation lake. Though scenic and undeveloped in all directions, even in the middle of summer (fondly referred to by the park locals as "the viewing season" instead of the "mud season"), the water temperature barely reaches a high of fifty degrees, so forays into the lake generally last less than a minute. Flowing out of the lake is the largest river in the park, the Yellowstone River. On most days, this wide waterway courses lazily northward, providing a haven not only for the abundant migratory waterfowl but also to fly fisherman slowly and delicately casting to rising brown or rainbow trout.

Sixteen miles to the north of the lake, the Yellowstone River has carved out a canyon that is eight hundred feet deep and twenty miles long. The two major park waterfalls, the Upper and Lower Falls, are easily viewed from places aptly named Inspiration Point, Artist Point, and Red Rock Point. A short hike from the road leads to an observation deck that is directly adjacent to the edge of the Lower Falls. The canyon's yellow and pink walls that are viewed from the deck vantage point led famous nineteenth-century painter Thomas Moran to proclaim, "Its beautiful tints [are] beyond the reach of human art."

Years later, I still vividly recall that toward the end of that very first day when I observed the Yellowstone Grand Canyon from the "Brink of the Lower Falls" viewing area, I felt deeply humbled by the reality of being in a location with landscapes like no other. I am always reminded that I was filled with a broader and deeper awe than just seeing nature's creatures. I opened my eyes wider, I breathed more deeply, and I felt warmth in my stomach. I imagined myself a pioneer exploring a newly discovered land, even though people armed with cameras, not old-fashioned rifles, surrounded me. I heard the gasp "Wow!" again and again as newcomers arrived at our viewpoint.

Throughout the park, I have learned over the years that there are forests untouched by logging, fields of subalpine and alpine wild flowers that grow without fear of future development, and a large variety of plants that grace the landscape in all directions and return each and every year with the turning of the seasons. There is even one forest made up entirely of petrified wood.

When the park was founded in 1872, the stated goal by the US Congress was "to create a park that [would] protect the natural magnificence of a unique area for future generations." During the "viewing season," the guests are truly sightseers experiencing Congress's wish, as Yellowstone and its habitat welcome them to a vast wonderland, though they are welcomed only transiently. In this manner, Yellowstone National Park is timeless. Though nature does evolve and change, in the park it largely does so without the weighty influence of human hands.

For most people though, a visit to the park ultimately revolves around a singular unique aspect of Yellowstone National Park. The park contains 10,000 thermal features, fully half of those that exist on the planet. Yellowstone is the home of geysers and mud pots and fumaroles. Yellowstone is the ageless and ever-changing home of boiling hot springs and multicolored travertine terraces.

A trip to a thermal area at Yellowstone might include the strange smell of rotten eggs, the sound of boiling water far from any stove, or the glorious sight of water blasting high into the air powered not by a fountain but rather the closeness to the surface of the earth's inner workings. The thermal areas awaken a different set of emotions than bison or jagged peaks; they are primal.

In the thermal areas, one is exposed to the immeasurable power of nature. Trees can be logged; rivers can be dammed; and animals can be captured, culled, or, in days long gone by, sadly exterminated. On the other hand, geysers emanate from the core of the planet and fumaroles spew steam over centuries not years.

For me, the park's thermal features inspire (and will always do so) unadulterated veneration and a sense of joy that I rarely feel elsewhere—except when my beloved Nancy is in my arms or lays asleep not far from me late at night. Only then can I hear the soft, rhythmic sound of her steady, quiet breathing as she waits for me to join her. Together we'll rise in the morning to face the day ahead—and all that a world filled with miracles and wonder will bring us.

About the Authors

Dr. Robert T. Winn is the long-serving medical director for the Deer Valley and Park City resorts in Utah. In this capacity, he administrates and sets policy for the on-mountain clinics that care for thousands of guests from around the world each year. For over twenty years, he also served as the medical director at the Old Faithful Clinic in Yellowstone National Park, the world's first national park, created in 1872.

In 2002, when Park City hosted the Winter Olympics, Deer Valley designated Dr. Winn its venue medical director in charge of all medical care for both athletes and spectators. Previously, in 1985, Dr. Winn acted as the overall medical director when Park City was the venue for the International Winter Special Olympic games.

Today Dr. Winn remains a long-term resident of Park City, Utah, and is also the cofounder of a large and diverse primary care practice that has grown to seventeen dedicated providers. He was born and raised in Wallingford, Pennsylvania, and completed his undergraduate studies at Pennsylvania State University, where he was a member of the Blue Key Honor Society and graduated Phi Beta Kappa.

Dr. Winn attended the Milton S. Hershey Medical School at Pennsylvania State University. While at Hershey, he received a foreign studies scholarship during his senior year to study in the rural town of Garkida, Nigeria. When he graduated medical school, he received the Gilbert S. Nurich award for scholastic excellence.

After discovering and falling in love with the mountains of the western United States, Dr. Winn chose to do his pediatric residency at the University of Utah in Salt Lake City, Utah.

His first job was as a solo physician at the Mammoth Clinic in Yellowstone National Park, where he met his wife, Nancy, to whom he has been married and deeply in love with for many years. He and Nancy have two children, Jayna and Jaret.

Dr. Winn remains very involved in the Park City local community and, at various times, has served several terms as president of the Summit County Health Board, as well as being a member of the Emergency Medical Services Council and a charter member of the Park City Educational Foundation Board. In his early years, he was the ambulance medical director when the ambulance service was all volunteers. Over the decades, Dr. Winn and his partners have provided medical assistance to the Sundance Film Festival, the Park City Ride and Tie, and the Autumn Aloft Balloon Festival. Dr. Winn's medical group has also served almost every local high school sports team and he has consistently and continuously participated in various school events, acting as chairman of groups such as Reality Town, Community of Caring, Great Books, and father-son events.

Dr. Winn was one of the founding members and early volunteers that helped staff the People's Health Center after Park City identified the need for a nonprofit health clinic for the uninsured and underinsured. When Park City was chosen as a finalist in the "All American City" national competition, Dr. Winn was sent to Cleveland by city leaders as a delegate for the final presentation. With a long-term commitment to community service, Dr. Winn has served as chairman of the "Children at Risk" committee that supervised the Park City Rotary Club's philanthropic activities with young people, in addition to many school and community activities.

Dr. Winn has received numerous accolades and public recognition for his work with park rangers, volunteer and professional ski patrollers, medical and nursing students, and medical residents from several different specialties and hospitals. He continues to enjoy showing students how to provide medical care like an "old-time country doctor." He treats his patients as family and knows them on a first-name basis, just as they know him by his nickname, "Winnie."

Dr. Winn's writing career is a direct outgrowth of his many years as a "teacher."

Timothy R. Pearson is the author of the number-one international and *New York Times* best seller *The Old Rules Are Dead*; president and CEO of The Thomas L. Pearson and The Pearson Family Members Foundation, the philanthropic intermediary of the Pearson Family that conceived and established The Pearson Institute for the Study and Resolution of Global Conflicts at the University of Chicago's Harris School of Public Policy Studies in September 2015; and founder, president, and CEO of Pearson Advisors ‖ Partners.

Pearson previously served as vice chairman, global managing partner, and first-ever chief marketing and communications officer for KPMG, the global Big Four accounting, tax, and consulting firm. He also was president and CEO of a leading international marketing and management consulting firm and, earlier in his career, he was president of several advertising agencies, where he led award-winning initiatives for leading global companies. He has received numerous global and national marketing honors and multiple awards, including *Advertising Age's* Best, Belding, Cable, Clio, Echo, Golden Phone, Lulu, Proto, PRSA Sunny, and the *Wall Street Journal's* Best.

He is also active with numerous civic and charitable organizations. In 2012 and 2013, he and his brothers Tom, Phil, and David were the first global benefactors of the Nobel Peace Prize Concert in Oslo, Norway, through The Thomas L. Pearson and The Pearson Family Members Fund. He has served on the Nobel Peace Center's advisory board and as a member of the Harvard Business School's Dean's Research Society.

Mr. Pearson graduated cum laude with a BA degree in English literature from DePauw University, where he was a Maxwell Scholar and president of Gold Key, the men's senior honorary society. He resides in Saddle River, New Jersey; Atlanta, Georgia; or Park City, Utah—depending on the temperature, the humidity, and the season.

About the Leukemia & Lymphoma Society

As the world's largest voluntary health agency dedicated to fighting blood cancers, The Leukemia & Lymphoma Society® (LLS) is leading the offensive to dramatically improve outcomes for patients with acute myeloid leukemia (AML), one of the most lethal blood cancers. LLS began funding AML research more than 66 years ago, and in the past five years alone we have invested nearly $100 million in AML research, with a focus on understanding the underlying causes of the disease to develop better therapies and save more lives. We are on the verge of realizing new hope for AML patients, who have not seen an advance in treatment in almost 40 years. LLS is uniquely qualified to change the landscape for patients with blood cancers, and other cancers, as we act as a catalyst for collaboration among medical centers, government, academia, and industry to advance the science on behalf of patients. Our mission is to cure leukemia, lymphoma, Hodgkin's disease, and myeloma and improve the quality of life of patients and their families. We fund lifesaving blood cancer research around the world and provide free information and support services for blood cancer patients seeking access to quality, affordable, coordinated care. Founded in 1949 and headquartered in Rye Brook, New York, LLS has chapters throughout the United States and Canada. To learn more, visit www.lls.org. Patients should contact the Information Resource Center at (800) 955-4572, Monday through Friday, 9 a.m. to 9 p.m. ET.